Energy Is Real! ™

A Practical Guide for Managing Personal Energy in Daily Life

Gail Christel Behrend

and

Claudette Anna Bouchard

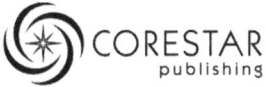

VANCOUVER, CANADA
energyisreal.com

2nd Edition Copyright © 2019 Gail Christel Behrend and Claudette Anna Bouchard

Cover design copyright © 2019 Bill Greaves (Concept West)
Cover art "Sun 2" by Bill Greaves (Used with permission)
Author photograph of Gail Christel Behrend by Lynn Landry
Author photograph of Claudette Anna Bouchard by Ashley Duggan (Keylight Photography)
Illustrations by Gail Christel Behrend

Published in Canada in 2019 by CoreStar Publishing

All rights reserved. Except for the inclusion of brief quotations in a review, no part of this book may be reproduced or transmitted in any form or by any means, without written permission from the publisher.

CoreStar Publishing

energyisreal.com

ISBN 978-0-9811937-1-7

Praise for *Energy is Real!*

"Outstanding! This highly informative and very practical book will teach you how to manage your energy so you can have the life you truly want for yourself. As a practicing clinician of 30 years, I consider this an absolutely must-have book for personal growth."
—Beverley Pugh, Registered Clinical Counselor, Vancouver BC, Canada

"*Energy is Real!* is a fantastic introduction for anyone wanting to learn more about this important and life-changing aspect of human life."
—Alexandra Amor, writer, Vancouver BC, Canada

"Claudette and Gail have done a masterful job in demystifying and exploring how to work with our own energy system. They teach us how to tap into one of our most valuable resources to promote health and well-being. Their book is filled with fun, easy and motivating self- care practices to incorporate into our daily lives. I highly recommend it for people who wish to live life to the fullest at any age!"
—Therese MacDonald, Registered Clinical Counselor, Surrey BC, Canada

"*Energy is Real!* is engaging and refreshing. It takes the reader on a journey of self-discovery through their energy bodies, with easy to understand language and exercises. I would love to have had this book when I first started to learn about the wonderful world of energy. This book can change your life! I will be recommending it to my clients and friends for sure!"
—Catherine Ralphs, RN, Vancouver BC, Canada

"Just like a manual for learning to drive, this book teaches you how to utilize and harness the vehicle of your own energy. It's fun, practical and very informative. Try it out!"
—Dr. S.A. McMurtry, Reiki Master, Vancouver BC, Canada

"I think this is a fabulous starter book for anyone wanting to learn more about energy and how to apply it in everyday situations!"
—Donna Evans-Strauss, Psychologist, Doylestown, PA

Acknowledgements

We wish to thank the following people without whose efforts this book would not have been published: Silvana Giesse, for her excellent coaching advice and editing skills; Bill Greaves, for an inspired cover design that so beautifully reflects our message; and Lynn Landry, for the author photos.

In addition, we wish to express our gratitude to our volunteer reader reviewers, whose support and invaluable feedback helped us to refine the book into its final form.

We also wish to thank the authors, teachers, coaches and mentors who over the years have provided guidance, training and inspiration to us on our individual journeys of transformation and growth. It is largely due to you that this book was written at all.

And last, but certainly not least, a big thank you to our clients, students, family members, and friends for encouraging us and helping us stay on course, one step at a time, as we learned about integrity, compassion, and being true to self through our experiences together.

Gail Christel Behrend
Claudette Anna Bouchard

Dedication

To my parents, Monica and Guenther. Your encouragement, patience and loving support are so appreciated.
> —*Gail Christel Behrend*

To my father, Butch and my mother, Germaine. Thank you for your love and support on this writing journey.
> —*Claudette Anna Bouchard*

Contents

INTRODUCTION XIII
   Why Read This Book? .... *xiii*
   What You'll Learn .... *xv*
   How to Use This Book .... *xviii*
   How to Access the Bonus Downloads .... *xix*

PART I: EXPLORING YOUR ENERGY NATURE

CHAPTER 1: THE WORLD OF ENERGY 1
   How Does Energy Affect Us? 3
      The Effect of Human Energy 3
      The Effect of Group Energy 4
      The Effect of Environmental Energy 5
      The Energy of Clothing and Objects 6
   Why is Energy Awareness Important? 7
      An Example—Energy Awareness Can Change Your Life 8
   How Do We Sense Energy? 13
      Consciously Sensing Energy 15
      Exercises to Explore Your Energy Senses 17
   Summary 28

CHAPTER 2: COMING HOME TO YOUR ENERGY SELF 29
   What Happens When We Lose the Self? 30
   How Do We Connect with the Self? 31
      Becoming Present in Your Body 31
      Becoming Present in Your Energy Field 33
      Creating a Strong, Safe Boundary 36
   How Do We Stay Centered While Interacting with Others? 38
      Managing Your Boundary to Deal with People or Situations 39
   Summary 44

CHAPTER 3: BECOMING CLEAR WITHIN 45
   Discovering Your Energy Self 46
      Exploring Your Physical Energy 47
      Exploring Your Emotional Energy 50
      Exploring Your Mental Energy 53
      Exploring Your Spiritual Energy 57
   How Do Your Different Energies Interact? 61
   What Stops Us From Expressing Our Energy Selves? 64
      What Happens When We Repress Physical Energy? 65
      What Happens When We Repress Emotional Energy? 66
      What Happens When We Repress Mental Energy? 68
      What Happens When We Repress Spiritual Energy? 69
   Summary 70

PART II: MANAGING YOUR ENERGY

CHAPTER 4: ENERGY AND SELF-CARE 73
   Why Do We Put Off Taking Care of Ourselves? 74
   How Does Neglecting Self-Care Affect Our Energy? 76
      The Effects of Neglecting Physical Self-Care 77
      The Effects of Neglecting Emotional Self-Care 77
      The Effects of Neglecting Mental Self-Care 78
      The Effects of Neglecting Spiritual Self-Care 78

Neglecting One Type of Energy Affects the Others 79
Why Make Self-Care a Top Priority? 79
    The Benefits of More Physical Energy 80
    The Benefits of More Emotional Energy 81
    The Benefits of More Mental Energy 81
    The Benefits of More Spiritual Energy 81
What Self-Care Do We Need for Better Energy? 82
What Do You Need Right Now? 83
Summary 87

CHAPTER 5: MAINTAINING YOUR ENERGY 89
   Conscious Breathing 91
    The Complete Breath 92
    The Calming Breath 94
    The Cleansing Breath...96
    Combining Breathing with Visualization 97
    Other Breathing Techniques 100
   Grounding (Connecting to the Earth) 101
    The Effects of Being Ungrounded 102
    How to Ground 103
    When to Ground 107
   Charging 111
    How to Charge Your Energy Field..112
    When to Charge Your Energy 117
   Clearing Unwanted Energies 118
    How to Clear Your Energy Field...119
    How to Clear Your Environment 125
    When to Clear Unwanted Energies 127
   Daily Energy Maintenance 128
   Summary 130

CHAPTER 6: SURFING YOUR PERSONAL ENERGY WAVE............................ 133
   What Happens When We Fight Our Energy?............................*134*
      Resisting Expansion...135
      Resisting Contraction 136
   Surfing Your Personal Energy Wave *137*
      Surfing the Peaks (Expansion Phase).................................137
      Surfing the Dips (Contraction Phase) 138
   Where Are You in Your Energy Cycle? *141*
   Summary..*143*

CHAPTER 7: RESTORING INNER BALANCE 145
   Balancing Your Physical Energy..*146*
      Physical Balancing Messages 147
      Restoring Your Physical Energy Balance 148
   Balancing Your Emotional Energy...*150*
      Emotional Balancing Messages 152
      Restoring Your Emotional Energy Balance 152
   Balancing Your Mental Energy *156*
      Mental Balancing Messages 156
      Restoring Your Mental Energy Balance 157
   Balancing Your Spiritual Energy *159*
      Spiritual Balancing Messages 160
      Restoring Your Spiritual Energy Balance 160
   Summary..*162*

PART III: TAKING YOUR ENERGY INTO THE WORLD

CHAPTER 8: ENERGY AND YOUR LIFE 167
   How Do Our Lives Get Out of Balance?................................*168*
   How Do We Know When Our Lives Are Out Of Balance? *170*
   How Can We Restore Balance in Our Lives?.........................*171*
      Self..172
      Abundance 173

    Communication 174
    Home and Family 175
    Play and Creativity 176
    Health 177
    Relationships 178
    Passion 179
    Learning 180
    Career 181
    Leisure and Social Life 182
    Purpose 183
How Balanced is Your Life? *184*
    Charting Your Life Balance 184
    Analyzing Your Life Balance Chart 186
    Restoring Balance in Your Life 189
Summary *192*

CHAPTER 9: QUESTIONS AND ANSWERS 193
  Questions on Chapter 1 The World of Energy *193*
  Questions on Chapter 2 Coming Home to Your Energy Self *196*
  Questions on Chapter 3 Becoming Clear Within *200*
  Questions on Chapter 4 Energy and Self-Care *203*
  Questions on Chapter 5 Maintaining Your Energy *208*
  Questions on Chapter 6 Surfing Your Personal Energy Wave *213*
  Questions on Chapter 7 Restoring Inner Balance *215*
  Questions on Chapter 8 Energy and Your Life *220*
  Taking Your Energy into the World *227*
  Summary *228*

FOR MORE INFORMATION 231
  Website *231*
  Join Our Facebook Group *231*
  Contact Information *232*

APPENDICES

Appendix A: Physical Balancing Messages 235

Appendix B: Emotional Balancing Messages 245

Appendix C: Mental Balancing Messages 255

Appendix D: Spiritual Balancing Messages 263

INDEX 275

ABOUT THE AUTHORS 281

Introduction

The study of human energy has been going on for thousands of years and many systems of health have developed around it, including traditional Chinese medicine, acupuncture, Ayurveda, homeopathy, energy healing, Tai Chi, Qi Gong, and yoga, among others. While these systems are now gaining wider acceptance, particularly in the fields of alternative health, most people generally don't understand how energy works or how to use it consciously in their daily lives.

Our aim in creating this book has been to demystify the subject of human energy and to show you how to manage your energy in practical ways that apply in today's modern world.

Why Read This Book?

After decades of personally seeing the effects of energy both in our own lives and in those of our clients, we know from direct experience that when people consciously manage their energy, they can create powerful changes in their lives. We've seen it happen many hundreds of times.

Benefits of managing your energy include:

- **Better health**—When you're able to restore energy flow to areas where you've repressed or frozen your energy, you can relieve pain or heal yourself of chronic illness. Energy techniques enable you to boost vitality, endurance and strength within minutes. You can also improve your mood or mental state quickly and easily by changing your energy.

- **Empowerment**—Being aware of energy, you're less likely to be deceived by those who try to manipulate you. You also have the energy skills to assert yourself effectively in any situation. When you understand the energetic implications of your actions, you make wiser decisions and become more accountable. Rather than blaming others, you begin to take responsibility for improving your own life.

- **Improved relationships**—By creating an energetic buffer of safety around you, you feel calmer and less anxious in relationship. You're able to honor your own needs, while respecting others. You feel safe enough to allow deeper intimacy with loved ones. Your positive energy makes you more attractive. Because your energy feels good to them, people are more likely to trust and support you.

- **Better work environments**—Energy skills can change conflict situations into creative win-win situations, improving your work life and relations with colleagues. Increased motivation, productivity, profitability, as well as improved morale and teamwork are sure to result.

- **More creativity and passion**—As you use your energy senses to explore the truth of who you are, you'll discover many of your previously accepted roles and beliefs to be false or limited. Once you open to your energy nature, you free yourself for more creativity and exploration. You have more passion and zest for life.

This book will teach you how to manage your personal energy so that you can experience these benefits for yourself.

What You'll Learn

Your body's physical senses of sight, hearing, taste, smell and touch bring you important information about your surroundings, but they do not tell you who you are. Your real sense of self comes from an inner awareness of your life force, feelings, thoughts, beliefs, memories, desires and ideals. You can't see these things, yet you know they exist and are what make you unique. In this book, we use the collective term "energy self" to refer to these subtle, nonphysical aspects of your being. This is the real self who thinks, feels and takes action in your life.

The purpose of this book is to help you to make the vital connection with your own energy self. As you do the exercises, you'll explore how various experiences affect your vitality and your sense of well-being. You'll discover that what you do with your energy affects every aspect of your life, including relationships with others. And you'll learn the basic techniques for managing your energy to create more health, happiness and fulfillment in your life.

The journey of getting to know and manage your energy has three parts. Here is a summary of what you'll learn:

- **Part I—This is the journey of exploring your energy nature:**

  - **Chapter 1,** *The World of Energy* describes common examples of how energy affects us in our daily lives, and provides exercises to sense energy in various ways. You'll discover that you probably already know more about energy than you may realize.

  - **Chapter 2,** *Coming Home to Your Energy Self* introduces you to your own energy field and teaches you how to connect with your real self. You'll also learn how to manage your energy to feel safe wherever you go.

  - **Chapter 3,** *Becoming Clear Within* explores your energy nature more deeply. As you delve within, you'll discover what you truly want and need in your life.

- **Part II—This is the journey of learning how to manage your energies:**

  - **Chapter 4,** *Energy and Self-Care* explores how neglecting self-care affects your energy levels. You'll also learn what self-care you need to keep your energies strong physically, emotionally, mentally and spiritually.

  - **Chapter 5,** *Maintaining Your Energy* describes four important techniques for building and managing your energies and provides practical exercises for applying them in your daily life.

  - **Chapter 6,** *Surfing Your Personal Energy Wave* explores how your energy moves in natural cycles. You'll learn how to work with your energy wave to best advantage.

  - **Chapter 7,** *Restoring Inner Balance* explores how to discover and interpret the balancing messages contained within your energy field. You'll also find out what actions to take to return to inner balance.

- **Part III—This is the journey of taking your new energy skills into the world:**

  - **Chapter 8,** *Energy and Your Life* explores how to create balance in your life, using the energy skills that you've learned in this book.

- **Chapter 9, *Questions and Answers*** provides answers to frequently asked questions about managing energy in different situations.

How to Use This Book

We've designed the exercises in this book to give you a direct experience of energy and to help you develop the necessary skills to manage your own energy in daily life. As you read each chapter of this book, we recommend that you take the time to do the exercises, so you can experience the benefits firsthand.

Because the skills build on one another, we suggest practicing each exercise until you become comfortable with it, before moving on to the next one. Your patience and diligence in the earlier exercises will reward you with more powerful insights and experiences later.

We also recommend that you keep a journal of your experiences with these exercises. Recording your experiences will teach you more about your energy every time you try the exercises.

Energy is real. We invite you to experience the truth of this for yourself. The sooner you can begin applying the techniques in this book, the sooner you'll be on your way to enjoying a healthier, happier and more rewarding life!

How to Access the Bonus Downloads

To help you to practice the skills and apply the concepts covered in this book, we offer free bonus audio MP3 recordings for all the exercises, as well as some worksheet PDFs.

In order to access these downloads, you will first need to register your copy of the book. You can do this by going directly to https://energyisreal.com/book/bonus-content, or by selecting *Book > Bonus Content* from the main menu on the energyisreal.com website.

As a registered book owner, you will also be eligible for additional bonuses as they become available. We will notify you by email when they are ready for download.

Please note that these materials are for your own personal use. We request that you do not share them with others without our express written permission.

PART I

EXPLORING YOUR ENERGY NATURE

CHAPTER 1

The World of Energy

Our energy weaves inextricably throughout the fabric of our lives. It's present in the unspoken communication that occurs between people, in the subtle shifts in power, in our maneuverings for attention and in the manipulative, comforting or inspiring currents that affect us in our relationships.

Here are some examples of common energy experiences:

- The realtor shows Anya into the next house on his list. As she enters, she starts smiling. This one feels like home.

- At a party, Fred finds himself cornered by a woman who carries on a long boring monologue about herself. The longer Fred listens, the more tired and drained he feels, yet somehow, he can't escape.

- Ellen, an elderly grandma, dearly loves small children, but feels exhausted after fifteen minutes in their company.

- When Bill's wife angrily demands an explanation for something he did, he can't find the words. His mind has gone blank.
- While running in a playground, five-year old Joshua trips and falls. His mother helps him up and kisses the bruise on his knee. Soon, Joshua feels much better and runs off again to join his playmates.

Our personal energy is not just something mysterious that we do or don't have; it is the life force and consciousness that inhabits our bodies. Our energy is an integral part of who we are and how we perceive the world.

At some level, we're all aware of energy in our lives. Our everyday speech frequently suggests this awareness, for example:

- "That boy has lots of energy."
- "I'm so in love! I'm walking on air!"
- "After arguing with him, I just have no energy left to face the day."
- "I worked on my taxes all day. I'm exhausted."
- "I am going to marry him. He's the one."
- "I can't explain it, but I have a strong feeling that she's lying."
- "I'm having second thoughts about this business deal. Something just isn't right."

In this chapter, we'll learn more about the world of energy and the benefits of energy awareness. At the end of this chapter, we'll explore sensing and playing with energy through a series of practical exercises.

How Does Energy Affect Us?

Energy can affect us positively or negatively. Negative energies leave us feeling fearful, upset or bad about ourselves. Examples of negative energy experiences include war, violence, pornography, witnessing a crime, mob behavior and toxic environments.

Positive energies, on the other hand, leave us feeling energized and uplifted. We typically feel good about ourselves afterwards. Examples of positive energy experiences include prayer, listening to beautiful music, giving and receiving love, walking in nature or appreciating beauty.

The Effect of Human Energy

We can all recall times when we've affected others with our energy and when others have affected us, for example:

- Our encouragement may have motivated someone to achieve a goal.
- We may have comforted a hurt child with a loving hug.

- We may have noticed ourselves getting tired and depressed when we were around someone who was in chronic pain.
- Prayer or singing may have uplifted us.

As we know from history, a single charismatic leader can move and influence thousands of people. Mahatma Gandhi, Martin Luther King and Adolf Hitler are just three examples that come to mind. Other more common examples include:

- A coach who motivates a team to win a game that they had been losing in the first half
- A gifted musician who moves an audience to tears through his performance
- A best-selling author who enthralls millions of readers with an imaginative story

The Effect of Group Energy

Group energy has a powerful effect on the energy of an individual. We're all familiar with the influence of peer pressure on the behavior of teenagers. Here is another example: when a comedian is in front of a receptive audience, he feels charged up and alive. Even his worst jokes evoke hysterical laughter. The next night, however, when the same comedian faces a "tough" audience of hecklers, his energy crashes and he struggles with every joke.

When people come together in groups, the effect of their combined energy multiplies exponentially. When strong feelings build within a group, it can cause people to behave in ways they would never act on their own. Riots, demonstrations, revolutions, crime and civil war are common examples of this phenomenon.

The energy of groups can also combine with positive results. For example, thousands of New Yorkers put aside their differences to help one another after the terrorist attack on the World Trade Center on September 11, 2001. As another example, when the 2004 tsunami hit Southeast Asia, the resulting devastation moved so many people around the world to help, that their combined donations exceeded the amounts offered by government foreign aid agencies.

The Effect of Environmental Energy

The energy of our environment (including homes, neighborhoods, workplaces, as well as natural surroundings) also has an effect on us. For example, how we feel downtown at rush hour is different from how we feel in a rural area. How we feel in a factory is different from how we feel in a church. And how we feel in our kitchen is different from how we feel in our bedroom.

Nature also affects us energetically. For example, storms can agitate or excite us. Rain can feel healing or depressing. Sunshine charges and energizes us. Sunsets calm us and can make us feel peaceful.

Conversely, we affect the energy of our environment. Human energy leaves its stamp. The occupants of a room imprint the walls and furnishings with their energy. This is especially true of emotional energy. For example, if a boss yells at someone in the conference room, the next group to use the room may feel unaccountably anxious or even irritable. Hospitals hold the energy of fear, stress, and anxiety from their patients and staff. That's partly why most people feel nervous and uncomfortable when visiting someone at a hospital. Battlefields, massacre sites and cemeteries also carry an energetic imprint, which sensitive people can sense.

The Energy of Clothing and Objects

Clothing and objects carry traces of their owner's energy. A thrift shop or used bookstore carries chaotic energy—to a sensitive person it feels like hundreds of people all talking at once. It's a well-known trick of pet owners to leave an old article of clothing in the pet's bed so their pet feels more secure while they are away.

Because we feel most comfortable in our own energy, many of us personalize the space where we work, no matter whether it is the executive suite, an office cubicle or a locker. We fill these spaces with our favorite pictures and objects, in effect leaving our own energy stamp on our environment.

Why is Energy Awareness Important?

When we have low energy, it's bound to affect our lives. Low physical vitality makes it more difficult to work or do what we love. When we don't have much emotional vitality, we feel burdened by the demands of our loved ones and may lash out at them—our relationships suffer. When our mental energies are low, we may feel confused and make poor decisions or we may defer to others to decide for us. When our spiritual energy is weak, we may feel a lack of purpose or direction. We may also feel bored or hopeless and despairing, or we may escape into drugs or alcohol rather than live our lives fully.

Conversely, when we're able to keep our energies strong and healthy, we find our lives improve dramatically. We have energy to spare. Our relationships become fun and joyful. Our love flows. Our minds are clear and decisive. Our sense of self expands and we find our creativity bubbling up with new ideas for self-expression. Life becomes exciting and meaningful.

Energy awareness is the first step to achieving health and balance. It helps us to sense where we're stopping the flow of our physical, emotional, mental or spiritual life force and how this leads to a similar imbalance in our lives. This larger awareness enables us to understand what changes we need to make to bring our energies and our lives back into balance.

Once we recognize the impact of the world of energy, we can learn the basic skills needed to take care of our energy fields so our health remains strong and vital. We can then also learn to manage our energy in daily life, so other people and external events do not throw us off balance as easily.

An Example—Energy Awareness Can Change Your Life

The story that follows will give you an idea of how being aware of your energy and knowing how to change it can improve your life, even when things go wrong. First, let's look at a typical "bad" day in the life of someone who doesn't know about energy. We'll call her Jane.

The Day from Hell

The alarm clock sounds at 6:30 AM. It's still dark outside. Jane's head pounds and her eyes feel swollen and gluey. The sound of rain drumming on the bedroom window does nothing to raise her spirits. She rolls over and burrows deeper under the covers, where it's comfy and warm.

An hour later, Jane wakes up with a start as she remembers that she has to give a presentation to management at 1 PM. She swears loudly as she looks at the clock. "7:30 AM! I am so late!" Leaping out of bed, she narrowly avoids tripping over the rug as she rushes to the bathroom.

Jane showers quickly and dresses. As she drags a comb through her wet hair, she looks into the mirror and sees dark circles under her eyes, still swollen from all the crying last night. Memories come flooding back of the fight with Andy, her boyfriend, correction, ex-boyfriend now.

Fighting back more tears, she glances at the clock. It is now almost 8 AM. She swears again. "No time for breakfast. I'll have to grab a muffin at break. I could stand to lose five pounds, anyway." Still putting on her coat, Jane rushes outside. As the house door slams behind her, she knows with a sickening certainty that she has just locked herself out. She's also forgotten her umbrella.

One tearful call to her neighbor later, she gets the spare key and runs inside to gather her belongings before dashing to the car. She is now extremely late.

The day doesn't improve when Jane gets to work. She snaps at her boss when he comments on her lateness and when he tells her the presentation to management has moved up to 10 AM, she has a full-blown panic attack.

Frantic, Jane tries to pull herself together to prepare her talk. Despite a growing headache, she manages to cobble together a slide presentation and finishes it just before the meeting. It looks hasty and unprofessional and she knows it. During the meeting, her mind keeps going blank and her boss has to keep prompting her with questions. What a nightmare!

Finally, with her presentation over and management's attention diverted to another speaker, Jane sneaks out and heads for the coffee shop downstairs. "Finally, something to eat!" Munching her muffin, Jane suspects that her day isn't going to improve any time soon. Her boss will certainly have something to say to her about that presentation, not to mention her snapping at him earlier. Then she'll have to face going home to an empty house—Andy won't be there to comfort her any more… The headache is rapidly turning into a full-blown migraine.

Well, you get the picture—who hasn't had a "Day from Hell"? But there's another way the day could have gone, had Jane known how to manage her energy. Let's take a peek at this alternate scenario.

The Power Day

As before, Jane wakes up feeling groggy and miserable. However, instead of rolling over when the alarm goes off, she sits up in bed and takes a long drink from the glass of water she has by her bedside. Thoughts of the fight with her boyfriend Andy fill her mind as she drinks. Tears begin to well up. Jane takes a deep breath to steady herself and starts with her morning check-in routine, starting with her physical state.

"My head aches. My sinuses feel stuffy and my eyelids feel swollen. I drank wine last night and cried a lot," Jane remembers, "I'm probably dehydrated." She drinks more water and soon notices her head beginning to clear.

Moving her awareness to her emotions, Jane thinks, "Whew! I feel like I've been through the wringer. Andy said he wants to see other people. That really hurt! I thought we were moving closer."

She spends a few moments just feeling her sadness and pain at the breakup, allowing herself to cry again. The ache in her chest and throat slowly eases with the tears. Jane decides to be kind to herself today. She gets up and makes herself some breakfast.

While eating her breakfast, she continues her check-in routine, tuning into her mental state. "My mind feels foggy and confused, with lots of thoughts milling around: 'I should have said this' and 'I wish I'd done that'."

Jane takes a few deep breaths and, counting slowly focuses on her breathing for a few moments. Her thoughts slow down and her mind becomes still; she is simply being present in the now. Her body relaxes.

From this quiet frame of mind, she shifts into her spiritual check-in.

"Who am I? And who am I without Andy? What am I doing with my life?"

In this state, Jane slowly realizes that for the past six months she has put her life on hold for Andy. She was writing a novel before she met him. Somehow, it had fallen to the wayside after they began seeing more of each other. "I want to start writing again," she thinks. She notices little flutter of joy inside her heart and begins to feel stronger.

Just then, Jane remembers the presentation to management due this afternoon. She grabs a pen and paper and starts jotting down thoughts that come to her as she eats her breakfast. Soon she has an outline for her presentation.

A glance at the clock reveals it's now 7:15 AM. Time to get ready. She moves purposefully, yet with a sense of kindness towards herself while she washes and dresses. As she combs her wet hair, she smiles at herself in the mirror, seeing a potential best-selling author looking back at her. "Today, when I get home, I'll start back on the book," she tells herself. The thought immediately cheers her.

It's time to leave, but Jane takes a moment to breathe deeply and become fully present. In that moment, she remembers to collect all her belongings, including her keys and umbrella, before leaving the house. Jane decides to take the bus today, so she can think about her presentation on the way to work. When she arrives at the office, she is smiling and ready to prepare the slides for her talk.

When her boss gives her the news that the meeting has moved up to 10 AM, she charges up her energy and shifts into productive gear to work on her slides. Since she has her notes from this morning, the slides don't take long to produce and when the meeting starts, she is ready and composed.

Jane takes another deep breath, and then visualizes being clear, concise and to the point. Her presentation unfolds exactly as pictured. She receives applause from management for her ideas. Buoyed by their approval, Jane spends a few minutes answering their questions at the end of the meeting. She feels calm, confident and collected. Management suggests several ideas and she ends up spending the rest of the day following up on them.

As Jane prepares to leave for home at 5 PM, her boss stops by her office to congratulate her on the presentation and drops hints about a job promotion for her. On this positive note, Jane heads for the bus. Noticing the rain has stopped, she decides to walk home. What a great day! Tonight she'll put on her comfiest clothes and begin working on her novel again. And if Andy calls? Well, that's what voicemail is for!

As you can see, our personal energy has a huge impact on how we experience and live our lives. Being able to sense and manage our energy gives us the ability to transform a "Day from Hell" into a "Power Day". Wouldn't you say that this might be worth learning?

How Do We Sense Energy?

We're all equipped with a complete set of energy senses that are just as real and as natural as our familiar physical senses. Ways that we can sense energy intuitively include:

- **Kinesthetically**—This energy sense is similar to the sense of touch or sensation. For example, we might notice the energy in a room feels heavy, sticky, stale, creepy, warm, tingly or even invigorating, depending on what just happened there.

- **Emotionally**—This energy sense evokes an emotional response in us. For example, we might experience the energy in a nursing home as a feeling of vague discomfort or fear. Conversely, the energy on a mountaintop can evoke a feeling of exhilaration.

- **Intuitively**—Our intuitive sense is a vague sense of knowing something, without any rational thought preceding it. For example, this occurs when we have a hunch who is calling us, even before we pick up the phone, or when we have a "gut feeling" that a particular opportunity or decision is right for us.

- **Inner hearing**—This energy sense feels like listening to our imagination. For example, a composer may hear inwardly the score of a new melody, containing all the various instruments and voices, which he then transcribes as musical notes on a page. Mozart is said to have composed this way. We may hear a calm inner voice encouraging us when we're down or we may hear and say exactly the right words that someone we love needs to hear from us.

- **Inner vision**—This form of seeing takes place in the "mind's eye", or mind screen, which is the same visual sense that we use in dreaming or imagining. If we have our physical eyes open at the same time, the energy vision superimposes over the physical vision. For example, we may see an aura of light around someone with colors that swirl and reflect their emotions.

- **Direct knowing**—This sense picks up detailed information about something, without any rational explanation. It is much more specific than intuition. For example, when thrust into a life-threatening emergency, we may become calm and somehow know exactly what steps to take. The urgency of the situation has caused us temporarily to open our awareness to the larger energetic picture, which allows us to make the right choices to save others or ourselves.

  Direct knowing is also the sense that receives specific details for a new idea, solution or creative project that suddenly occurs to us while we're doing something unrelated, like driving or taking a shower.

- **Love**— We sense the energy of love deep in our hearts. Love is more than just an emotion. Love is a nourishing energy that has powerful creative and healing properties. Works of music, poetry, art and writings inspired by love transcend the boundaries of nationality, race or time—they still affect us centuries later.

Consciously Sensing Energy

Most of us notice energy in subtle ways as something that just "happens" to us. However, we can also consciously use our energy awareness in practical ways, just as we would use physical sight to search for lost keys or use physical hearing when tuning a car radio to a favorite station. For example, you can use your energy awareness to detect danger. Gail relates her first experience of using her "energy radar" as follows:

"Many years ago, I had come home from work to find my front door unlocked. I couldn't remember whether I had locked it that morning and I was scared that a prowler might have broken in and was waiting for me inside. What to do?

"I wished that I could somehow pour my mind through the keyhole into my apartment and check for an intruder while staying safely outside in the hallway. 'Well, why not try it,' I thought. So, I allowed my awareness to enter and fill the entire apartment. My sense was that everything was normal and that no one was in there.

"For some reason, I trusted this impression. I cautiously entered my apartment, keeping my awareness open wide. I explored each room to appease my logical mind. The place was untouched, as I had sensed. That was my first experience of consciously trying to sense energy."

You can also use your energy awareness to find your friends in a crowd or at a mall. Gail relates the following experience of trying this:

> "I had agreed to meet a friend at the International Jazz Festival in Vancouver. We had left the arrangements vague. We both wanted to see different performers at the same time and agreed to meet in David Lam Park afterwards. Of course, during the jazz festival thousands of people crowded the park. How was I going to find my friend? If he had a cell phone it would have been easy, but he refused to own one.
>
> "I stood still and closed my eyes. Then I tuned my awareness to search for his energy—it felt like looking for a blip on a radar screen. In my mind, I sensed his energy far away and to the left.
>
> I walked about fifty yards through the crowds in that direction and then checked again. Ah! He was moving. Now, I sensed him straight ahead, but still far away. I walked forward for another fifty yards or so and checked again. I sensed him closer, but over to the right somewhere.
>
> I saw a path a few yards ahead veering off to the right, so I wove through all the people and turned onto that path. Suddenly I heard "Hey Gail!" And there was my friend!

Once we know how to sense energy, we begin to discover many practical uses for energy awareness in our daily life. Over time, our energy senses become automatic and normal. Our sense of self and our experience of life become fuller as we become more aware of what's going on energetically within us and around us.

Exercises to Explore Your Energy Senses

Although it's possible to sense energy in any or all the ways described earlier, we tend to use the senses that are most comfortable to us, our preferred energy senses. With practice, we can learn to expand our energy horizons by developing all our inner senses. This section provides some exercises that you can use to explore how you personally sense energy.

Sensing Energy with Your Hands

For most people the easiest energy sense to connect with is the kinesthetic sense. Here are some simple exercises for kinesthetically sensing energy with your hands:

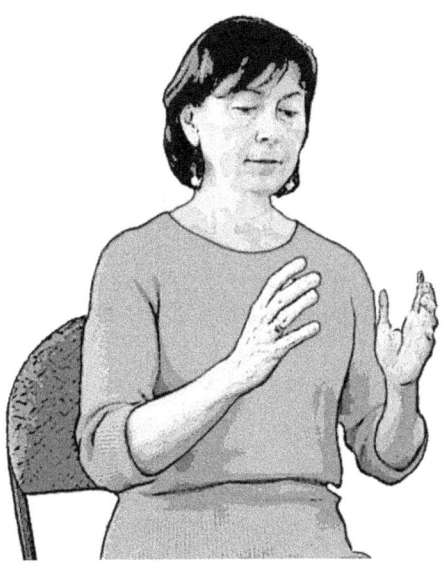

Exercise 1-1 Sensing Energy with Your Hands

Exercise 1-1: Sensing Energy with Your Hands

Have paper and pen handy to record notes.

1. Sit in a comfortable position.

2. Bring both of your hands together, palm touching palm and fingers touching fingers.

3. Rub your hands together until they become hot from the friction. This charges your hands.

4. Then, allow your hands to float gently apart to wherever they want to be. Stop there and simply sense your hands. What is the energy like between them?

5. Move your hands toward each other. What do you sense? Then, let your hands float apart to where they want to be.

6. Move your hands farther apart from each other. What do you sense? Then, let your hands float back to the neutral position.

7. Experiment with moving your hands back and forth to sense how the energy changes.

8. When finished, drop your hands and rest comfortably.

9. Record your experience in your notes.

You can also try this exercise with a partner.

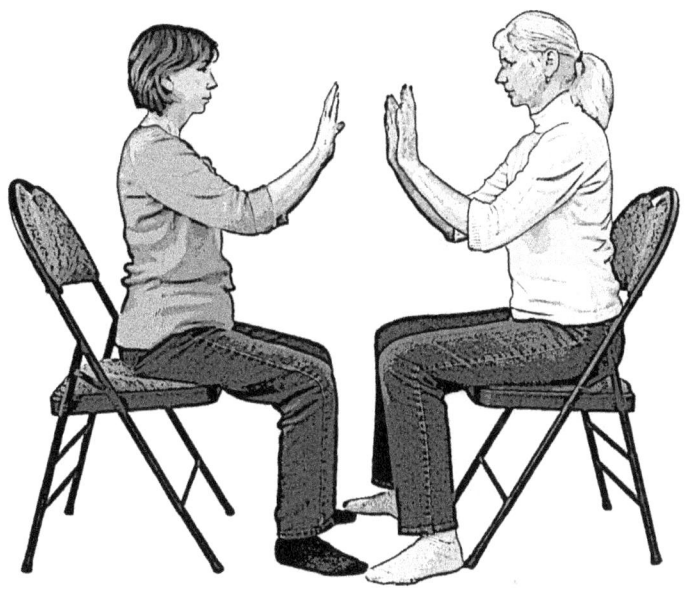

Exercise 1-2: Sensing a Partner's Hands

Exercise 1-2: Sensing a Partner's Hands

Have paper and pen handy to record notes.

1. Sit in a comfortable position facing each other.

2. Rub your hands together (as in Exercise 1-1) and hold them up with your palms facing your partner's palms.

3. Move your hands toward your partner's hands until you sense something. What is the energy like between your hands and your partner's hands?

> 4. Move your hands toward your partner. What do you sense? What does your partner sense?
>
> 5. Move your hands farther away from your partner. What do you sense? Do you notice any difference? What does your partner sense?
>
> 6. Ask your partner to move their hands closer and farther away from you, while you hold your hands still. What do you sense?
>
> 7. When finished, drop your hands and rest comfortably.
>
> 8. Record your experience in your notes.

Sensing Your Energy Field

All life forms, including humans, have energy fields, which are not visible for most people, although we can sense them in other ways. For example, we instinctively know what our own energy feels like. We know where our energy ends and someone else's energy begins. When we're sitting on a park bench with our eyes closed, and someone sits beside us, their energy feels different from ours.

We also have an intuitive sense of how much space we need to feel comfortable. Everyone has had the experience of someone standing too close to us. When this happens, the person is standing partially inside our energy field. It's as if we carry our private territory around with us. People have different standards for how much personal space they need to feel safe. Some people keep their energy fields close to their body. Others need several feet of space around them to feel comfortable.

Most of us are able to feel this space intuitively, kinesthetically or emotionally (as a sense of threat or safety). If your inner vision is sensitive, you may also be able to see it as an aura of light around yourself or others.

The following exercise will help you to sense your energy field.

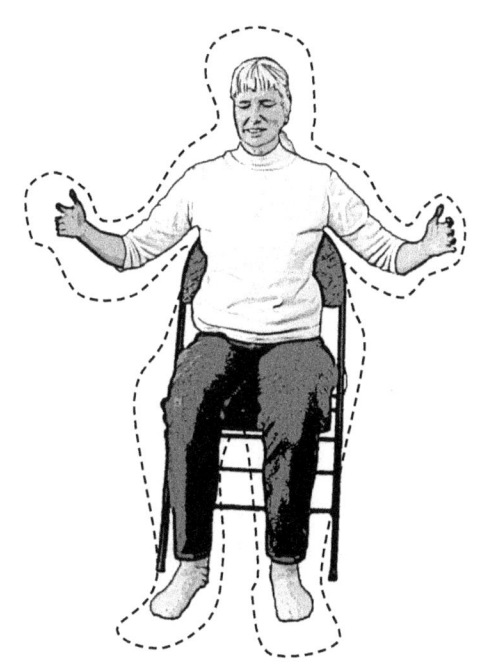

Exercise 1-3: Sensing Your Energy Field

> ### *Exercise 1-3: Sensing Your Energy Field*
>
> Have paper and pen handy to record notes.
>
> 1. Sit in a comfortable chair and close your eyes.
>
> 2. Take in a long, slow, deep breath and let it out with a sigh.
>
> 3. Take another slow breath and as you breathe in, feel your body sitting on the chair. If your body is in discomfort, change your position until it feels comfortable. Release your breath with a sigh.
>
> 4. Continue to breathe slowly and become aware of your own life force. Feel its energy down to the bottom of your feet on the floor, up to the top of your head, and around the sides of your body.
>
> 5. Notice how your energy field feels. Does your energy feel close to your body or more extended out from your body? How far out does it go?
>
> 6. Try bringing the energy closer in or extending further it out. Play with it. Notice in what position your energy feels most comfortable. Is it farther away or closer to your body?
>
> 7. Record your experience in your notes.

Changing the Boundary of Your Energy Field

The energy field, also called an aura, reflects where our sense of self extends and how much room we need around us to feel safe. This aura, which extends below our feet, can expand or contract depending on the situation and on how we feel. The outer edge of the aura is called a *boundary*.

In the following exercise, you'll explore changing the boundary of your energy field.

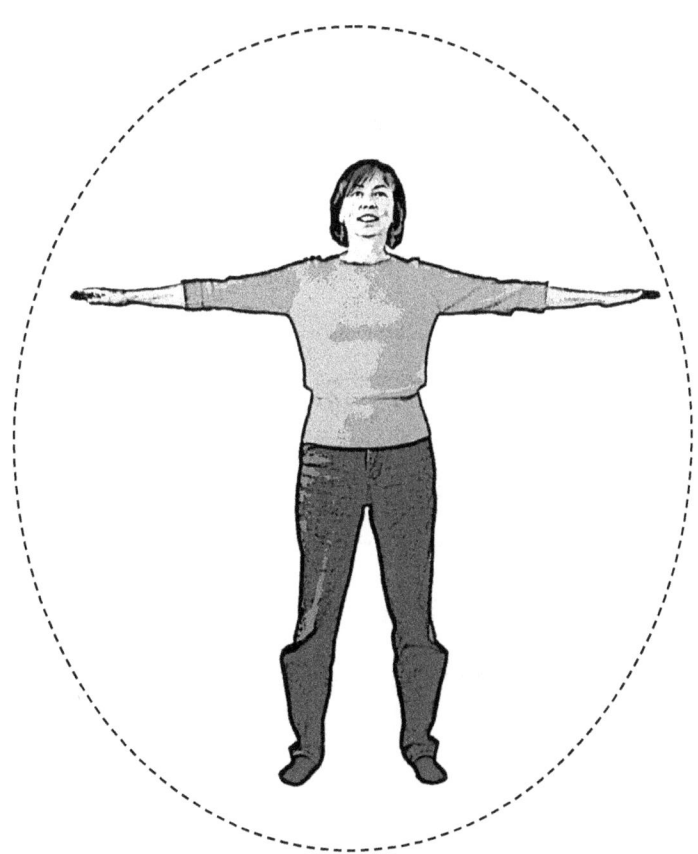

Exercise 1-4: Changing the Boundary of Your Energy Field

> ### *Exercise 1-4: Changing the Boundary of Your Energy Field*
>
> Have paper and pen handy to record notes.
>
> 1. Standing straight, stretch your arms out to the sides of your body, then out to the front, then out to the back and then above your head.
>
> 2. Allow your aura to extend out to your fingertips, all around you, above you and below you. The area marked out by your fingertips is the boundary of your energy field. Try to sense what your boundary feels like in this position.
>
> 3. Now imagine shrinking your boundary inwards to your elbows all around you. Notice the difference.
>
> 4. Return your boundary to a comfortable position. Record your experience in your notes.

Sensing Other Peoples' Boundaries

When people are moving about in a crowd, sometimes their fields will touch or even overlap your energy field. Below is an exercise that you can do with a partner or a group of your friends to experience this. You can also quietly try this exercise next time you go someplace where there are other people, such as in a mall or at a party.

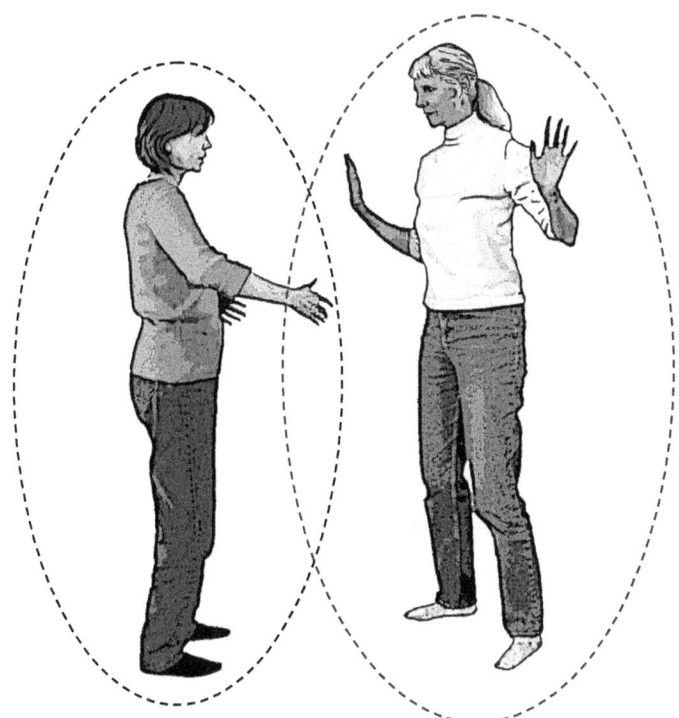

Exercise 1-5: Sensing Other Peoples' Boundaries

Exercise 1-5: Sensing Other Peoples Boundaries

Have paper and pen handy to record notes.

1. Gather a group of friends together or go to a public place where there are other people.

2. Walk around the room, passing near one another.

3. Notice how you feel when someone is in your field and when you're alone in your field. Can you tell where their field begins and yours ends?

4. Record your experience in your notes.

Sensing the Energy of Places and Objects

The following exercise will give you a direct experience of how places and objects affect you energetically.

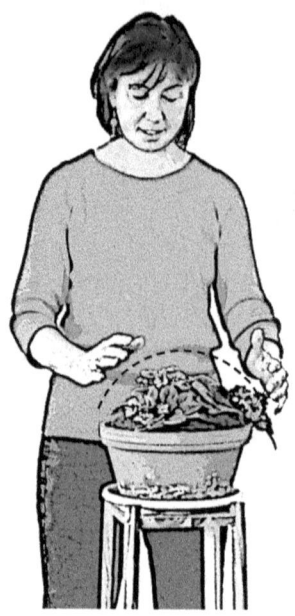

Exercise 1-6: Sensing the Energy of an Object

Exercise 1-6: Sensing the Energy of Places and Objects

Have paper and pen handy to record notes.

1. Sit or stand in a comfortable position indoors.
2. Close your eyes and feel the energy of the room. Notice how your energy reacts to sounds or other sensory distractions.

3. Notice your thoughts and anything that might be coming up in your imagination. What is your experience of being in this environment?

4. Open your eyes and look around the room. How does your energy react to visual distractions, objects and beauty?

5. Walk around the room. What is your experience of being in different parts of the room? Where do you feel drawn to go? Where do you feel safer? Where do you feel less safe?

6. Sense the energy of different objects. Explore the energy of houseplants, furniture, clothing and personal objects like wristwatches or jewelry. What differences do you notice?

7. Go outside and explore different spaces in Nature. What is your experience?

8. Explore different buildings, for example: your office, a public library or a thrift store. Which places feel better than others? Which places feel uncomfortable to you? How do they affect you emotionally or mentally?

9. What did you learn? Record your observations in your notes.

Your Primary Energy Senses

Review the list of energy senses beginning on page 13. Based on your experiences with the previous exercises, what are your primary energy senses? Record your observations in your notes.

Summary

In this chapter, we learned about how our personal energy responds to the energy of other people, places and objects, as well as our own thoughts and feelings. We also explored how to sense energy in different ways. If you tried the exercises in this chapter, you've had a direct experience of how your own energy feels and what affects it. You may also have drawn some conclusions about your preferred way of sensing energy.

Like many other worthwhile skills, the fastest way to develop your energy awareness is through practice. Try the exercises given in this chapter with your friends. Make up some new energy games or exercises. Have fun with it! Here are some you could try:

- Play with sensing energy at the bank, at work (it makes meetings more interesting!) or in school, for example.

- Feel the energy of different places. How does a church compare with a bus station?

- Try it outside in Nature. How does the energy in a garden compare with the energy in a forest?

Now that you've had some experience sensing the world of energy, it's time to learn more about your own energy nature. In the next chapter, you'll begin a deeper exploration of your own energy and you'll learn some practical techniques that will help you to feel safe wherever you go.

CHAPTER 2

Coming Home to Your Energy Self

Most of us do not consciously recognize or make full use of our energy nature. Imagine how much richer life would be if we were to engage all of our senses, including our energy awareness, rather than limiting ourselves to just our physical senses, our linear intellect and our reactive emotions.

When we pay attention to what our energy is telling us, we begin to discover our true selves. We begin to notice what works for us and what doesn't. We learn how to respond to the external world in a way that reflects who we really are. We take ownership of what makes us happy and what doesn't. We begin to choose decisions that lead to happiness. Hope grows in us as our love expands to include ourselves as well as others. It's powerful. The old saying, "Know thyself," begins to make sense.

Our inner world is calling us to pay attention, to open the door and to cross the threshold to experience more of ourselves and more of what life has to offer. In this chapter, we'll open that door and help you to find the way back home to your energy self.

What Happens When We Lose the Self?

When we forget what is important to us, when we lose touch with our own needs, priorities, dreams, values and ideals, we've lost our sense of self. As a result, we tend to defer to others and find ourselves rushing around to fulfill the demands of other people, while neglecting our own needs.

For example, let's say somebody asks us to organize something. We automatically drop everything and rush to do it, without thinking. Later we ask ourselves "How did I get talked into doing that?" It's because we lost our sense of self in that moment.

Here is another example: we're at a pub with our friends and somebody buys a round of beers. Then someone else buys a round. Soon everyone is taking turns buying rounds. We might not want to continue drinking, but the peer pressure is on—they are all saying "come on, have another!" If we don't have a sense of self, we'll continue. Instead of saying "no," we're swept along with what's going on and ignore our own need to stop.

Or else, we're trying to quit smoking. We haven't smoked in three weeks. We go for coffee with an attractive co-worker who offers us a cigarette. To be sociable we accept it. The next thing we know, we're back to smoking a pack of cigarettes a day. How did that happen? We lost our sense of self.

When we're in touch with ourselves, we take the time to pause and check within whether we really want to do something or not. We may have many reasons why we can't or don't want to do it right now. So, before agreeing to something, we first check with ourselves to see if it works for us in that moment. We may still choose to do what someone asks, but because it's a conscious choice and not automatic, we also accept responsibility for our actions and are willing to accept the results.

How Do We Connect with the Self?

We connect with ourselves through a process called *centering*. Centering involves three steps:

1. We bring our conscious awareness fully into the body.
2. We extend our awareness to include our energy field.
3. We create a strong energy boundary, or energy bubble.

This section describes each of these steps in more detail.

Becoming Present in Your Body

When frightened or threatened by something, many of us partially leave our bodies energetically. When this happens, we feel lost, scattered and unsure of who we are. We don't know what to do next. We're like deer frozen on the spot by headlights. In extreme cases, we may even pull our energy so far out of our bodies that we lose consciousness and faint.

When we leave our bodies energetically, our logical minds don't know what to do. It's only when we return our energy to our bodies, that we're able to bring ourselves back to the present moment and harness our minds to deal with whatever situation is confronting us.

Becoming present in the body is a skill well worth learning. With practice, it eventually becomes an instinctive response to stress, which greatly helps us to deal with difficult situations or people.

The following exercise is especially useful when our thoughts are circling about in the past or future and we're not aware of what is happening around us. When we take the time to breathe consciously, just being mindful of our breathing and paying attention to our physical sensations, it brings us back into the body and into the awareness of here and now. When we're able to change the state of our awareness from mentally preoccupied to physically present, we've learned a basic and most crucial energy skill.

Becoming present in the body requires focusing on the breath and at the same time becoming aware of our body sensations. Exercise 2-1 describes the steps.

Exercise 2-1: Becoming Present in Your Body

Have paper and pen handy to record notes.

1. Stand or sit with a straight spine.

2. Take slow deep breaths—about six seconds to fill your lungs and six to empty them.

3. Bring your awareness to your breath. When breathing in, feel the air coming in through your nostrils, down into the lungs and then

> imagine the breath moving into all the cells of the body. As you breathe out, feel the lungs emptying and the air flowing out through your nostrils.
>
> 4. Repeat about five or six times until you become aware of your whole body, from your head to your feet.
> 5. Explore your physical sensations, the weight of your clothes on your skin, wiggling your toes, noticing the floor pressing against the soles of your feet.
> 6. Lean left and right, back and forward, noticing how your weight shifts over your feet or in your chair.
> 7. Now open your other senses: hearing, sight, taste and smell. Let the other senses wash over you while staying present in your body. If you get distracted, focus on your breathing to bring you back.
> 8. Record your experience in your notes.

Becoming Present in Your Energy Field

If you did the exercises in Chapter 1, *The World of Energy*, you discovered that your sense of self extends out to a certain distance from the body. It seems to have definite edges—it feels like a capsule or bubble around you, defining the boundaries of your personal "comfort zone". This is your energy field.

We unconsciously expand or contract the boundaries of our energy field depending on who we're with and on the situation. For example, we may like to snuggle up close with our loved ones or our pets, but feel we need more space with strangers or people who intimidate us.

The size of our energy field also varies according to what is normal for our culture. People in some cultures prefer closer physical proximity than those in other cultures, and this different sense of personal space can lead to misunderstandings. Because it's an energetic phenomenon, people may not even be aware that their different personal boundaries are causing stress in a relationship and subtly fueling a lack of trust between parties.

In addition to the size of the field, the boundaries of the field may be thick or thin, intact or broken, flexible or rigid. Some people have such porous boundaries that they have difficulty distinguishing themselves from others. These people are often extremely sensitive to energy. It may be painful for them to be around loud or emotional people. They may feel very unsafe in their bodies. They may often react defensively towards others, because everything feels like an invasion to them. We call them "thin-skinned".

Conversely, someone with a strong inflexible boundary may seem completely impervious and insensitive to others. Insults and arguments bounce right off them. Our language calls them "thick-skinned".

The self extends beyond the body into the energy field. So, to connect fully with who we are, we need to become present in our energy fields as well as our bodies. Exercise 2-2 describes the steps.

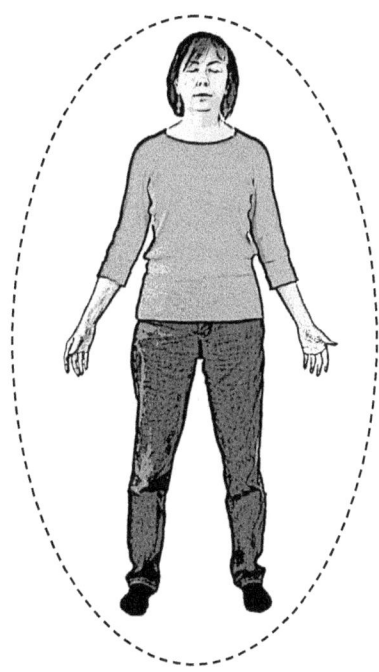

Exercise 2-2 Becoming Present in Your Energy Field

Exercise 2-2: Becoming Present in Your Energy Field

Have paper and pen handy to record notes.

1. Stand or sit with a straight spine.
2. Follow the steps in Exercise 2-1 to bring your awareness fully into your body.
3. As you relax into your body, notice how being present gives you a warm comfortable feeling in your body. Let yourself breathe into that warm feeling a few times, letting the breath expand it.

4. Now breathe deeply into that warmth and allow your sense of self to expand beyond the body, past your skin and into the space around your body. Let that warmth expand all around you as far out as you can reach to fill your entire field.

5. Allow yourself to relax all the way into this warm expanded sense of self. It is all you. Notice how much space you need to feel comfortable. Relax into it. Claim that space for yourself by filling it with your energy.

6. Record your experience in your notes.

Creating a Strong, Safe Boundary

Our sense of self and our energy field unconsciously expands or contracts depending on how safe we feel. When we don't feel safe, fear contracts our energy inwards—we feel small and vulnerable. When we do feel safe, our hearts open and our energy expands.

Love is the highest energy frequency. When we're in a loving state, we're able to see others and ourselves with more compassion. We feel clear, empowered and strong. We can access our heart's wisdom—an inner sense of knowing about what is right for us. We're able to feel our own worth. We rediscover our natural gifts and abilities. In essence, we're able to access our highest and truest expression of self.

When we consciously fill our energy fields with loving energy, it strengthens us to deal effectively with what is going on for us in our lives. It creates a solid foundation of safety and trust within us. And when we feel safe and secure, then the people and events of our lives are less likely to knock us off balance.

The following exercise describes how to create a strong, safe boundary around your energy field. This is your personal "energy bubble".

Exercise 2-3: Creating an Energy Bubble Around You

Have paper and pen handy to record notes.

1. Stand or sit with a straight spine.
2. Bring your awareness to your breath. Feel the breath relaxing your body, mind and spirit. Relax into your self and rest for a moment in the warm comfort of your own energy.
3. When you feel comfortable, expand that sense of comfort to that perimeter that extends to the end of your fingertips all the way around you, so your energy fills your field.
4. When you can feel your energy surrounding you, allow your awareness to move into your heart area.
5. As you rest in your heart, open your awareness to the feeling of love. If you have trouble feeling love, just remind yourself of somebody you love or a cherished pet.
6. Allow that beautiful feeling of love to expand spherically to fill your field all the way out to the boundary. Keep filling the field with love until the boundary feels firm and strong. This is your energy bubble. Notice how it feels to be in your bubble right now. This is your space, your safety, your world.
7. Record your experience in your notes.

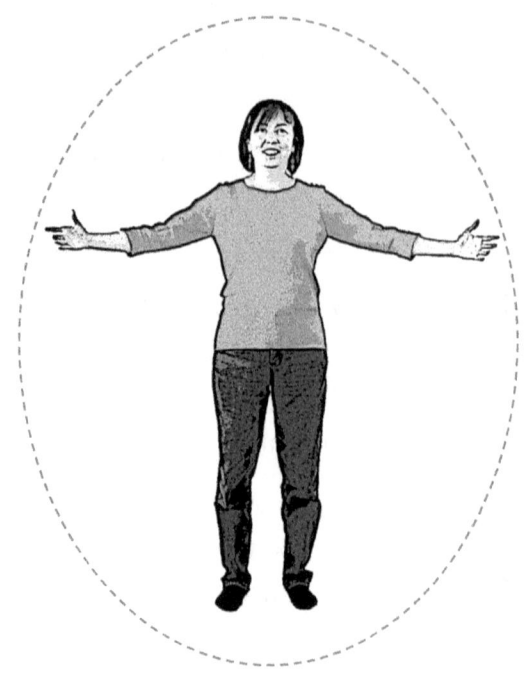

Exercise 2-3: Creating an Energy Bubble around You

How Do We Stay Centered While Interacting with Others?

Once we're fully present in our bodies and our energy fields, and we've created our energy bubbles around us, we feel centered, at home. We start to get a sense of what makes us feel good, what doesn't make us feel good. We have something to work with. When we've experienced that sense of safety, we want to be in that place all the time.

However, external events and other people can cause us to become uncentered. They trigger our emotions, which causes our energy to react and then we lose our sense of self. If we're uncomfortable in any given situation, it tells us that our boundaries have become weak; our energy bubble is not in place. Our energy has shrunk from our fields and we're most probably hiding out in our heads. When we retract our energy to our heads, our bubble deflates, so it's easy for someone to influence us, because there is no energy inside holding the boundaries out. So how do we deal with the external world?

Managing Your Boundary to Deal with People or Situations

When we fill our field with love, the field becomes strong with firm boundaries—like a fully inflated balloon. It takes practice, but when we're able to hold the boundaries of our field with our awareness, the energy of other people slides off the sides of the field, rather than invading us. We're holding our own space.

So, by staying in our hearts and filling our fields with love, we can interact more effectively with other people. Our firm, but loving boundary keeps them from controlling us.

Exercise 2-4 will help you to experience the truth of this for yourself.

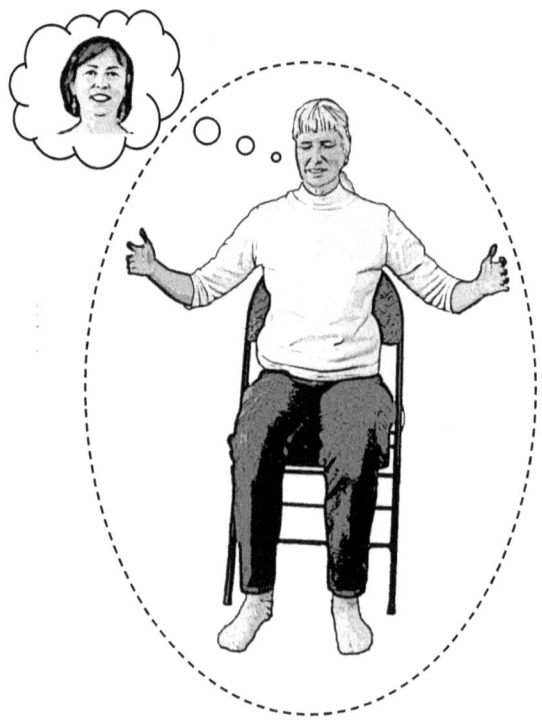

Exercise 2-4: Managing Your Boundary to Deal with People or Situations

---

Exercise 2-4: Managing Your Boundary to Deal with People or Situations

Have paper and pen handy to record notes.

1. Stand or sit with a straight spine.
2. Take a few deep breaths and follow the breath inwards until you're relaxed and fully present in your body (see Exercise 2-1).

3. Expand your awareness into the rest of your energy field until you feel fully present in your field (see Exercise 2-2).

4. Move into your heart and create that beautiful feeling of love. Allow it to expand throughout the whole field to create your energy bubble (see Exercise 2-3). Notice how it feels to be in your energy bubble right now.

5. Now, move your attention to the edge of your field. Imagine somebody with whom you're having difficulty communicating, and with whom you'd like that relationship to be different. It could be a spouse, a colleague, a friend or a family member— anybody with whom you're having a hard time.

6. Notice how your field automatically responds to that thought. If you've noticed that your field has shrunk in, that's fine, leave it where it is, but imagine that person outside your field. Still keeping that person outside the field, let the love in your heart expand again to inflate the bubble.

7. Keeping that person outside the field, imagine how you would like your relationship to be with this person. Notice how your bubble responds.

8. Look at that person outside your field. How do they look to you now?

9. Record your experience in your notes.

If you did this exercise, you may have noticed that a positive change occurred in the other person. Perhaps they started smiling. While you were imagining the best relationship, you were evoking the energy of love. When this happened, the other person responded to the love you radiated in your field. This is all energetic! You've just changed the dynamics between yourself and that person. That person is no longer controlling you energetically or emotionally. Why? Because you've created space for yourself.

You can use this exercise to develop your skill in managing your boundaries before taking it out into the real world. Explore a variety of scenarios, with different people or imagined situations. What's the dynamic?

If your field contracts, or feels wobbly and uncertain, it means that you're not feeling safe within yourself when you think about a person or situation. So, fill your field with love again and place that person or situation outside the bubble where they belong. Notice how much easier it is to relate to them when you keep them outside your boundary and provide that space for yourself.

We don't even have to imagine changing the situation. Just putting them outside our field and inflating our energy bubble again with love, helps us to become more comfortable with the situation. We don't need to look around for solutions. What's important is how we feel inside ourselves. When we create that calmness and safety within, we're able to act more wisely in a situation.

Our bubble provides automatic safety. We don't have to think things through. We don't have to analyze. We're so full of that high frequency energy of love that we can trust ourselves to do and say the right thing automatically. This creates a strong foundation for interacting with people.

Some of our clients have asked, "You know when I have that bubble up, it feels like a shield—it feels like it separates me from other people. But I don't want to turn people away. How can I keep my sense of self and still let people in?"

The answer is that we can have our bubble and we can let people in. But we let people in with our hearts, not our heads. When we're in our hearts and we expand loving energy to fill our entire field, then we experience a fuller sense of self. As soon as we leave our hearts and retract our energy to our heads to interact with the other individual from our minds, then our bubble collapses.

Our culture, our upbringing and our experiences have taught us that we have to protect our hearts and only interact from our minds. But the bubble allows us to be able to interact from both our hearts and our minds, and still have that sense of wholeness and safety.

It is also important to realize, that we don't have to leave our hearts to be able to think or communicate clearly with others. We can expand our awareness to include our whole energy self—body, heart, mind and spirit. Not only does it make us feel safer and stronger with others, it also provides us with more inner resources for dealing with daily life situations. Later in Part III, we'll explore how involving your energy self in all areas of your life will help you to deal more effectively with the external world.

Summary

In this chapter, we explored how to connect with the self. We learned how to center ourselves in the energy self, first by becoming physically present in the body, then by extending our awareness into our energy fields and finally, by strengthening the boundaries of our fields to create an energy bubble for ourselves.

It takes time to train ourselves to claim and hold our space. We need to keep practicing and honing our skills. When we feel uncomfortable, we can stop blaming the environment, the situation or the people around us. We can let go of analyzing. Instead, we can ask ourselves "Am I in my bubble right now?" If the answer is no, then before we do anything else, we get our bubble back in place again. That will help us to deal more effectively with the situation.

When we're consistently able to create a strong boundary for ourselves, we can be anywhere in the world and still feel safe. Then we're ready to go inside our energy field to explore who we are and what we need, unaffected by other people's demands and expectations.

In the next chapter, we'll learn how to do this and in the process, we'll meet our real self. We'll discover how to become clear within ourselves.

CHAPTER 3

Becoming Clear Within (Who Am I?)

When we pay attention to how our energy responds in everyday circumstances, we learn how our habits and choices affect our energy levels. Knowing this, we can begin to make better decisions in our lives.

We start treating others and ourselves with more kindness, not to be nice or because we "should' do this, but because we've discovered that loving energy feels great!

We've experienced for ourselves that love actually increases our vitality. And we've learned that love evokes more cooperative responses from those around us. As a result, our lives begin to flow more smoothly and gracefully. We become joyful, creative and alive.

Connecting with the real self is about finding our own rhythm. It's about discovering what gives us joy and pleasure, and what choices make the best sense for us as individuals. Finding our rhythm helps us to get rid of self-doubt and to find harmony within.

In this chapter, we'll explore what goes on inside our energy fields and we'll experience how our thoughts, emotions, beliefs and our physical energy levels all interact.

Discovering Your Energy Self

What is your experience of your self, right now? What does your energy feel like? What's happening now inside you? What's important to you? What do you want for yourself? What do you need right now? All of these questions explore who you really are in this moment. At any given time, you can check inside yourself to see how you're feeling physically, emotionally, mentally and spiritually.

Until you connect with what is important to you, you'll never be completely happy in your life. Exploring your real self is a journey through varied landscapes—the different parts of your being.

Some of these aspects may be very familiar, such as body aches or pains, your feelings towards others and your reactions to how they treat you. Other parts of your being may be less familiar to you, such as your thoughts, dreams or beliefs.

Some territories may even be largely unexplored, such as the subconscious patterns governing the choices you make in your life and the reasons you react the way you do in relationships.

As you go even deeper, you'll also explore spiritual themes such as "Who am I?", "What is my life about?", "What am I doing here?" and ultimately "What is going to fulfill me?"

Exploring Your Physical Energy

Physical energy is most familiar to everyone. We all know immediately when we feel drained of physical vitality, for example, when we drag ourselves out of bed on a Monday morning. Most of us have also experienced plentiful vitality at some time in our lives, even if it was only during childhood.

We may have also learned from experience how our overall health affects our physical energy levels. For example, when we're suffering from the flu, we feel tired and achy and we just don't have the energy to do all that we normally do when we're healthy.

Our physical energy affects how much we can do in our lives. But, as well as reflecting the amount of vitality or life force we have, our physical energy sensations also provide us with important messages about how we're living our lives. Symptoms such as tension here, tightness there, cold sweat, prickles or rapid breathing all tell us that something is amiss.

When we're fully present in our bodies and energy fields, we become aware of these inner messages. And we can use them as signposts pointing to where we need to make changes in our lives to return to balance and health.

Check-In Exercise to Explore Your Physical Energy

What is your experience of your physical self, right now? You can use the following check-in exercise to explore the state of your physical energy.

Exercise 3-1: Exploring Your Physical Energy

Have paper and pen handy to record notes.

1. Find a comfortable position and close your eyes.
2. Bring your attention to your breathing.
3. Take in a deep breath and let it out with a sigh. Repeat this 3 times.
4. Allow your awareness to tune into your physical body. What is your overall physical vitality like right now? Is it high (lively), medium (relaxed) or low (tired), for example?
5. Take another deep breath and let it out with a sigh. Allow your awareness to sink even deeper into the body.
6. Ask yourself the following questions:

    - Where is my energy right now? Am I all the way in my body or am I only partially occupying it? Is my energy flowing freely or does it feel stuck somewhere?
    - Is my energy balanced front and back, left and right?
    - What sensations am I aware of?
    - Which parts of my body are calling for my attention right now?
    - What is my general level of comfort?
    - What is my body wanting me to do right now?

7. When finished, take another deep breath and let it out with a sigh.
8. Open your eyes and record your experience in your notes.

Doing this exercise provides a quick snapshot of the state of your physical energy in the moment. Our physical energy is not static, however. It is constantly changing and responding to what is going on in our lives.

To get a fuller picture of what influences your physical energy, try doing this check-in at different times and under different circumstances every day. For example, try it on waking in the morning, at work, on the weekend, after exercise and before going to sleep.

Record what you find in your energy journal. Try to gather data for a week. What did you learn about your physical energy self from this exploration?

Check-in Examples

Here are a few physical check-in examples:

- "My physical energy feels low. My neck is stiff and I feel tense, especially just below my stomach. I feel a need to relax outside, maybe take a walk on the beach this afternoon."

- "My energy is sleepy and I'm getting hungry. When I check deeper, the first thing that gets my attention is my lower back—it feels sore and a bit cold. I need to eat, drink more water and get more fresh air. I really want to dance, too—music is a great way to boost my energy!"

- "Physically, I feel great—I have loads of energy! I have been working out three times a week. I really notice the difference in my energy levels compared to six months ago. Checking deeper, though, my attention goes to my abs, which feel sore. I think I overdid it yesterday doing my crunches. My body wants me to take it easier today. Also, I could drink more water. I feel dehydrated."

Exploring Your Emotional Energy

Our emotions are also part of our energy field. Humans can experience a vast array of emotions. Some of our emotions, like grief or jealousy, can be extremely painful or distressing. Other emotions, like gratitude and joy for instance, are very enjoyable.

We can direct our emotional energy outwards or inwards. When we yell at others in anger, for example, it can feel like a force hitting them. When we're feeling sad, remorseful or guilty, our emotional energy moves inwards.

We may describe emotional energy as having sensations, temperatures or textures. For example, anger feels hot—we call someone who angers easily "hotheaded" or say they have a "fiery temper." Love feels warm and light. Despair, sadness or grief feels heavy and liquid—we say people are "drowning in sorrow". Bitterness may feel cold and hard, "His heart turned to ice."

Some people can sense emotional energy as having a color. We even reflect this in the English language, when we use such expressions as "feeling blue" (sad), "seeing red" (angry), "green with envy", "in a black mood" (despair) or "having a sunny personality" (cheerful).

Check-In Exercise to Explore Your Emotional Energy

What is your experience of your emotional self, right now? You can use the following check-in exercise to explore your emotional energy.

Exercise 3-2: Exploring Your Emotional Energy

Have paper and pen handy to record notes.

1. Find a comfortable position and close your eyes.

2. Bring your attention to your breathing.

3. Take in a deep breath and let it out with a sigh. Repeat this 3 times.

4. Allow your awareness to go inward and tune into your emotions. What is your overall emotional vitality like right now—high (passionate), medium (calm), low (flat or numb)?

5. Take another deep breath and allow your awareness to sink even deeper into your emotional energy.

6. Ask yourself the following questions:
    - What is my general level of emotional comfort?

- Which emotion is calling for my attention right now?
- Can I safely express this emotion right now, or later when I am alone?
- If I can't express this emotion, where does it go? What happens to this energy when I don't express it?

7. Repeat step 6 for any other emotions that you're aware of right now.

8. When finished, take another deep breath and let it out with a sigh.

9. Open your eyes and record your experience in your notes.

Try doing an emotional check-in under different circumstances during the day, especially when you feel uncomfortable or stressed about something. For comparison, also do a check-in when you're feeling happy or balanced.

Notice how various circumstances and people affect you emotionally. Record what you find in your energy journal. What did you learn about your emotional energy self from this exploration?

Check-In Examples

Here are a few emotional check-in examples:

- "I don't feel much emotional energy right now. I feel kind of flat or even bored. As I go deeper, actually, I do notice some discomfort. It feels like anger or resentment. It's not something I feel safe to express right now. I'm holding it in my stomach, like a tight fist."

- "I feel emotionally vulnerable right now. I had a fight with my boyfriend last night and we both said some hurtful things. I'm feeling sorry right now about what I said, even though it was true. I am afraid that our relationship may be over. I feel a mixture of fear and sadness in my heart area."

- "My emotional energy feels high. I feel upbeat and positive about the changes I am making in my life. I feel strong and confident. I feel excited about my promotion at work and the business trip to Paris coming up next week!"

Exploring Your Mental Energy

Our mental energy includes not only our thoughts, but also our ability to think clearly, to reason, to analyze, to focus and to plan. It includes our intuitive mind, our memories, knowledge, techniques and skills that we've learned, as well as our ability to communicate clearly with others.

Our mental energy is an important aspect of our energy self. We can change our overall energy levels in an instant just by changing our thoughts. We do it all the time. For example, we're feeling great one moment and then we run into an old acquaintance who tells us about some wonderful experience, for example falling in love or getting a new sports car.

Although we may act happy for our friend, inside we suddenly feel our energy has fallen through the floor. One moment we feel great, the next terrible. What happened here?

What probably happened is that we had a thought such as "I'll never be able to do that," or "He has all the luck" or made some other unfavorable comparison. Comparing thoughts are often self-judging. And self-judgment drains our energy. We do it so automatically that we're typically not aware of even thinking those thoughts. All we know is that suddenly we feel low or flat.

The more we think about how bad we feel, the worse we get. If we allow our thoughts to focus on all that is wrong in our lives, we can easily fall into a negative spiral of gloom. Then we fail to see the many opportunities around us that could improve our lives.

Conversely, when we think about our achievements or when we think lovingly toward ourselves or others, our energy increases. We feel energized and more able to take action. We become more positive and attractive, so more opportunities come toward us. For example, in the "Power Day" story in Chapter 1, when Jane thought about getting back to writing her novel again, it gave her a positive boost of energy and confidence that carried her forward for the rest of her day. For these reasons, it's worth paying attention to our mental energy states and noticing how they influence our lives.

Check-In Exercise to Explore Your Mental Energy

What is your experience of your mental self, right now? You can use the following check-in exercise to explore the state of your mental energy.

Exercise 3-3: Exploring Your Mental Energy

Have paper and pen handy to record notes.

1. Find a comfortable position and close your eyes.
2. Bring your attention to your breathing.
3. Take in a deep breath and let it out with a sigh. Repeat this 3 times.
4. Allow your awareness to go inward and tune into your thoughts. What is your overall mental vitality like right now? Is it high (quick), medium (thoughtful) or low (sluggish), for example?
5. Take another deep breath and allow your awareness to sink even deeper into your mental energy.
6. What is the state of your mental energy in this moment? Ask yourself the following questions:

    - How clear is my thinking?

    - Am I able to focus or concentrate? If not, what is distracting me?

    - Where are my thoughts going? Here and now? In the past? In the future?

    - How capable am I of objectivity? Am I judging others or myself?

- Am I thinking logically or intuitively?
- How easily can I communicate my ideas and thoughts to others in this moment?
- Am I able to make wise decisions right now?

7. When finished, take another deep breath and let it out with a sigh.
8. Open your eyes and record your experience in your notes.

A good time to do a mental check-in is just before you need to make a decision. Find out if your current mental state is conducive for making the right choice for you, and if not, give yourself some time before deciding. As soon as you can, make sure your bubble is in place. This will provide you with the space to collect your thoughts.

Use the mental check-in exercise to explore how various circumstances affect you mentally. Notice also how your mental state affects your communication with others.

Record what you find in your energy journal. What did you learn about your mental energy self from this exploration?

Check-In Examples

Here are some mental check-in examples:

- "Mentally, I feel slow and groggy right now. I drank too much alcohol at the party last night and have a hangover. Now would not be a good time to make any important decisions. Even trying to think hurts. All I want to do is just go home and sleep it off."

- "My mental energy feels strong and quick. My thinking is clear and focused. I had some great ideas this morning and want to keep going while I am on a roll. I have a report to get out this afternoon, so I feel pressured, but it's nothing I can't handle."

- "My mental energy feels chaotic. My thoughts are all over the place and I'm having trouble getting focused. I keep reliving the argument I had with my boss earlier. 'I should have said this,' 'I should have said that,' and so on. I know I have to get organized, but I can't seem to pull my thoughts together."

Exploring Your Spiritual Energy

Our spiritual energy includes our dreams, creative impulses, a sense of destiny or fate, inspiration, joy, love, values, ethics, conscience, a sense of purpose and our inner wisdom—the promptings and stirrings of our soul. If we follow these inner promptings, we find our lives filled with joy, delight and purpose. This can happen at any age.

That part of our spiritual energy that we call our conscience is based on our ethics, morals and values. If we follow a religion, our conscience may reflect the beliefs and creed of our chosen faith. If we don't follow a religion, our conscience may reflect our philosophical or cultural beliefs, or simply what we learned from our parents.

Our spiritual energy is the source of our creativity and our inspiration. It communicates with us through our dreams, through our imagination or through an inspired idea that appears out of nowhere. For example, we may be taking a shower and suddenly think of a creative solution to a problem that has been nagging us.

Or we may have a sense that something is guiding or encouraging us, for example, we may think we hear the voice of a beloved grandparent. We may think it's just our imagination, but we're strangely comforted anyway. If we follow the guidance, we discover to our amazement that it's exactly what we needed to do. Wherever it came from, it's through our spiritual energy that we're able to receive this information.

Our spiritual energy also works the other way—we can create visions as well as receive them. For example, we may daydream about our future success as a best-selling novelist, imagining our next novel published and in the bookstores. This is a powerful ability. When you picture what you want to create, your spiritual energy then begins to attract those opportunities, ideas and people who are in energetic harmony with your vision.

Check-In Exercise to Explore Your Spiritual Energy

What is your experience of your spiritual self, right now? You can use the following exercise to explore the state of your spiritual energy.

Exercise 3-4: Exploring Your Spiritual Energy

Have paper and pen handy to record notes.

1. Find a comfortable position and close your eyes.
2. Bring your attention to your breathing.
3. Take in a deep breath and let it out with a sigh. Repeat this 3 times.
4. Allow your awareness to go inward and tune into your spirit. What is your overall spiritual vitality like right now? Is it high (expanded), medium (peaceful) or low (depressed), for example?
5. Take another deep breath and allow your awareness to sink even deeper into your spiritual energy.
6. Ask yourself the following questions:
   - Who am I? What is important to me?
   - Am I living in alignment with my values and ideals?
   - Do I feel connected to and supported by life?
   - What creative ideas and inspirations are coming up for me right now?
   - How do I feel about myself and the world?
   - Am I living in a meaningful way?
   - What is my heart telling me right now?
   - What are my dreams telling me?
7. When finished, take another deep breath and let it out with a sigh.
8. Open your eyes and record your experience in your notes.

Ideally, you want to do a check-in of your spiritual energy in a place where you can be alone and free from distractions for a few minutes. For example, you might do a check-in when you first wake up, while taking a bath or shower or just before going to sleep. If possible, try to remember your dreams—they may have important messages for you from your own spirit.

Begin to note how the state of your spiritual energy affects your outlook and your effect on others. Also, pay attention to the coincidences that occur in your life. See if there is any connection with the themes that you're noticing in your spiritual check-in.

Record what you find in your energy journal. What did you learn about your spiritual energy self from this exploration?

Check-In Examples

Here are some spiritual check-in examples:

- "On the spiritual level, my energy feels good. I guess I would give my overall spiritual vitality a rating of medium. I feel grateful for my life and all the things I have achieved. My creativity is flowing and I'm excited about the poetry I have started to write. It feels inspired. I'm also grateful for my wonderful wife. She truly feels like my soul mate. We connect on so many levels. I feel happy and fulfilled."

- "Spiritually, I'm feeling on the low side, right now. I feel down about my girlfriend leaving me. She accused me of dabbling in life, not committing myself to anything. Maybe she's right.

What have I got to show for the last 20 years? Sure, I've had fun, but it feels like something's missing. What do I really care about? What do I want to spend my life doing? I don't know. But I feel an inner longing to find out. Also I have a nagging suspicion that I shouldn't put it off too long."

- "My spiritual energy feels very high. I just finished a weeklong retreat meditating in the mountains. I feel so connected with everything and so supported right now. I have a sense of deep certainty that I'm finally on my right path. It's only been a month since I decided to open a center to help children with AIDS in my community. Already financial donations are just pouring in. I am so excited about this!"

How Do Your Different Energies Interact?

Our physical, emotional, mental and spiritual energies are not isolated from one another. They exist as part of a greater whole—our energy self. Our sense of self pervades all aspects of us and our energies reflect that wholeness. What happens to one part of our energy also affects all the other parts.

Low physical vitality, for example, will drag down our emotional, mental and spiritual energies. That's why when we're sick, we're more likely to feel irritable or depressed and we're more likely to think pessimistic thoughts. Also, we're more likely to feel helpless about our recovery.

On the other hand, if a loved one sends us flowers or cheers us up in some other way, then that positive energy boost will move through the other parts of our field. Soon, our mental outlook improves and our physical energies increase to speed our healing.

Exercise to Explore How Your Energies Interact

Everyone's energy self is different, because our bodies, emotions, thoughts and beliefs are different. No two people will react identically to the same events. Try the following exercise to discover how your own energies interact and reflect your unique energy self.

Exercise 3-5: Exploring How Your Energies Interact

Have paper and pen handy to record notes.

1. Find a comfortable position and close your eyes.
2. Bring your attention to your breathing.
3. Take in a deep breath and let it out with a sigh. Repeat this 3 times.
4. Allow your awareness to go inward and tune into your physical body. What part of your body is attracting your attention right now? Notice the first physical sensation that comes. For example, you might sense tightness in the upper back.
5. Take another deep breath and allow your awareness to sink into that part of the body.

6. Tune into the emotional energy in that area. What emotions are you feeling there? Notice the first emotion that comes into your awareness. For example, you might feel burdened or unsupported in the upper back area.

7. Tune into your mental energy in the same area of your body. Ask yourself what thoughts might be causing that emotion. Notice the first thought that comes into your awareness. For example, you might get the thought "I'm tired of having to clean up after everyone else."

8. Tune into your spiritual energy in that area of your body. Ask yourself what beliefs you might be holding that are causing those thoughts. Notice the first belief or conclusion that comes into your awareness.

    For example, you might notice a belief that says, "I am the responsible one. Everybody else gets to have fun, while I do all the chores." Notice if there is a particular childhood memory that arises as you explore your belief.

9. Now change your spiritual energy by imagining a scenario where the opposite belief is true. For example, if you feel burdened, imagine being on vacation instead. There is nothing for you to do except enjoy yourself. Vividly imagine all the ways you would have fun.

10. Do a physical, emotional and mental check-in. Notice how imagining that scenario has affected your thoughts, emotions and physical sensations in that part of your body.

11. When finished, take another deep breath and let it out with a sigh.

12. Open your eyes and record your experience in your notes.

Try this exercise a few times with different types of physical symptoms.

Or, instead of changing your spiritual energy as in step 9, try changing your mental energy—choose a different thought or attitude. See what that does to your energy, physically, emotionally and spiritually.

Make a change to your physical energy—take a walk or do some yoga stretches, for example. How has the change in physical energy affected your thoughts and emotions in the problem area?

Sometimes, despite all attempts, you may feel you're unable to budge the symptom or the associated emotion, thought or belief. If this is the case, then you may be stopping or repressing your energy physically, emotionally, mentally or spiritually in this part of your energy self.

What Stops Us From Expressing Our Energy Selves?

When we express our energy selves naturally and easily, we're able to experience vibrant health, emotional happiness, mental clarity and spiritual fulfillment. If we're dissatisfied in any of these areas, chances are that we're stopping ourselves from fully expressing some parts of our energy.

Why do we stop ourselves? Usually it's because we think it's not safe to express those parts of ourselves. The reason may be subconscious—buried in some long-forgotten, painful childhood experience. Or it may be conscious, for example, religious or cultural taboos or our childhood upbringing may forbid that form of self-knowledge or self-expression.

What Happens When We Repress Physical Energy?

When it causes us discomfort to express our physical energy in some part of our body, we may unconsciously repress our energy in that area. For example, if some part of our body is in pain, we may avoid using that area of the body. And we may divert our energy away from that place to prevent ourselves from feeling the pain.

Sexuality is natural part of our physical expression, but many people block their sexual energy. Some people stop their sexual energy because they find sex physically painful, or they have uncomfortable beliefs about sexuality. Others may repress their sexual energy because it brings up painful memories of childhood abuse. Members of a religious order may hold back their sexual energy because they have taken a vow of celibacy.

Regardless of the reason, when we repress our physical energy, we unconsciously block it from flowing. When we block it, it has nowhere to go and begins to stagnate in the place where we're blocking it.

Areas in the body downstream of the block starve from lack of energy. Over time, physical problems may develop in the affected areas, because the underlying cells are energetically undernourished.

In Chapter 7, *Restoring Inner Balance*, you'll discover where in your body you block or repress your physical energy and you'll learn how to move your physical energy so you can quickly return to balance again.

What Happens When We Repress Emotional Energy?

Our ability to express emotions depends on our childhood upbringing and culture. And some emotions are easier for us to express than others.

For example, many men find it easier to express anger than sadness. When experiencing sadness, a man may not recognize the emotion for what it is. He may think that he is simply tired or angry.

Women, on the other hand, are often more comfortable expressing sadness than anger. When experiencing anger, they may turn it inwards rather than directing it at someone else. Then when they turn the energy inwards, they may feel sad or hurt instead.

When we repress strong emotions, such as anger or grief, it lowers our energy levels all around. Eventually, we can't experience joy or pleasure in our lives anymore. We become lethargic and depressed. We may take prescriptions to boost our emotions artificially or to calm ourselves so we can cope. We may spend years in psychoanalysis trying to figure out what is wrong.

But what is really happening is that we've learned poor energy habits—we hold back those troublesome emotions instead of expressing them in a healthy way.

If we learned to fear anger when we were children, then as adults we may be unable to express anger in healthy ways. For example, we may contain our anger for so long that we don't recognize when we're angry anymore. Then one day, a minor upset happens, and we suddenly explode. Our reaction is out of proportion to the triggering event.

This is similar to what happens with a garden hose. When we shut off the water flow at the nozzle, the water pressure builds in the hose. Then if we open the nozzle again, for a few seconds the water jets out forcefully until the pressure subsides and the flow returns to normal.

The healthy expression of anger does not need loud outbursts. If we state our position clearly and firmly when we first become angry, then our emotional energy flows normally and resolves itself. We become able to act to improve the situation.

Our best approach to dealing with our emotions is to look at them as just forms of energy. When we understand that for health, our emotional energy needs to flow, we can learn to express our emotions naturally, without self-judgment and without social embarrassment.

Energy management skills can help to move emotional energy in safe ways, with no harm to others or ourselves. In Chapter 7, *Restoring Inner Balance*, you'll learn some techniques to work with your emotional energy so you can quickly return to balance again.

What Happens When We Repress Mental Energy?

As with emotional energy, we can also repress or block mental energy. For example, when we worry excessively and our thoughts go in circles with no resolution, we experience a *mental impasse*, where we can see no way out of the situation.

The circling thought pattern becomes frozen in the energy field—we can't decide so the energy gets stuck. Because we don't allow any fresh mental energy in, we can't receive any new ideas that could solve the problem.

We may have a communication problem that we feel unable to resolve in our relationship and rather than deal with it, we may choose to ignore it. When we ignore the problem, it doesn't go away; it stays in our field until we're able to address it.

If we continue to detour our attention away from the problem, our mental energy has no chance to be released. Over time, the stuck energy becomes a block, which causes problems in the emotional and physical parts of our lives.

Unexamined thoughts keep us feeling overwhelmed and confused. But by consciously examining our thoughts, we have the option to replace them with empowering thoughts and beliefs, allowing our mental energy to flow freely again.

Chapter 7, *Restoring Inner Balance* describes techniques for unblocking and uplifting your mental energy so you can keep your mental abilities healthy and strong.

What Happens When We Repress Spiritual Energy?

If we ignore or repress our inner promptings, our spiritual energy freezes and our lives eventually feel shallow and meaningless. Living with an uncomfortable conscience also robs us of peace of mind and prevents us from being able to relax and enjoy our lives fully. The constant inner stress drains us of energy.

When we ignore or repress our spiritual energy, over time it can lead to physical problems. Often it affects the spine (e.g. misalignments), heart (for example pain or palpitations) or head (for example headaches, problems with eyesight or hearing).

It can also lead to emotional problems such as depression and despair. And it can affect us mentally, creating a sense of confusion and indecision about life. We may use food, drugs, alcohol, workaholism, or even shopaholism to avoid feelings of despair and lack of meaning in our lives.

When we live out of alignment with what is important to us spiritually, we're betraying ourselves at a deep level. This betrayal erodes our trust and confidence in ourselves, which eventually leads to unconscious self-sabotage. If we find ourselves unable to take the necessary steps towards some cherished dream, chances are we have a spiritual energy block affecting some area of our lives.

Chapter 7, *Restoring Inner Balance* describes some techniques for opening to the gifts, abilities and wisdom contained within your spiritual energy so you can bring joy, direction and a sense of purpose into your life.

Summary

In this chapter, we learned about the four kinds of energy that make up our personal energy self. We learned how to bring our awareness inside the field and sense the physical, emotional, mental and spiritual levels of our being.

If you've been practicing these exercises, you'll have directly experienced your own energy nature and begun to get to know your real self.

In Part II, you'll learn how to read your energy so you can find out what you need to get your life back into balance. You'll also learn new skills to manage and maintain your energy day-to-day.

PART II

MANAGING YOUR ENERGY

CHAPTER 4

Energy and Self-Care (How Can I Feel Better?)

Many of us are so drained by stress that we often don't have enough energy left for the activities and people we care about. Our lives feel out of balance and we don't know what to do about it.

Restoring and recharging our energies happens naturally when we follow the wisdom of our body and life force. So, why are so many of us exhausted and tense? It's because we've lost contact with that inner wisdom and as a result, we've forgotten how to take care of our own energy.

Energy awareness ensures that we pay attention to the things that are important to our happiness and well-being, *while they are happening*. Proper self-care ensures that we have ample health and vitality to make good decisions, take suitable action and fully appreciate our lives as they unfold.

In this chapter, we'll explore what stops us from taking proper care of ourselves and how this affects our energy levels. We'll also learn how to sense what self-care we need to keep our energies strong on all levels of our being—physically, emotionally, mentally and spiritually.

Why Do We Put Off Taking Care of Ourselves?

Why is it so hard for most of us to take proper care of ourselves? Why do we put it off, even though we know it will lead to a healthier, more enjoyable life?

Here are some common reasons we neglect self-care:

- **We resist authority, even our own**—Some of us subconsciously resist anything prefixed with a "should." We steadfastly refuse to be "told what to do", even by our own conscience. We resist any kind of authority on principle.

- **We feel self-care is selfish**—Many women and some men hold the subconscious belief: "I must always put other people (especially children) first, otherwise I'm being selfish." When we hold this pattern, we feel that self-care is stealing time and energy that we should spend on helping others. Self-care is only acceptable after we've done all our "chores" and have taken care of everyone else.

- **We think self-care is weak**—Those who are extremely competitive may consider self-care only in terms of physical exercise, possibly even as a demonstration of achievement: "I spent 3 hours working out at the gym yesterday—just look at these abs!" or "I'm preparing for a marathon. Look at me!" But even as they're training, these people are likely to overdo it. They're out of touch with their body's real needs, including the need for enough rest and nourishment. As soon as a competitive mood crops up, self-care is the first thing to go. The prevailing thought is, "Self-care is for wimps! I'm tough!" Such people are more likely to strain a muscle and to ignore the warning messages their bodies give them.

- **We believe self-care is boring and restrictive**—Some people equate self-care with self-deprivation, for example, having to eat a restricted diet, doing hard exercise, or giving up late night parties and social drinking. They may be afraid their friends will judge them as boring. Their belief is "Who wants to be healthy, if it means you have to give up the fun in your life?"

- **We think self-care is a luxury**—Many people, on the other hand, confuse self-care with self-indulgence. But self-care is not the same as self-indulgence. Self-indulgence is what happens when we neglect self-care. It's a form of escape that's not nurturing. While it may feel good in the moment, the effects are short-lived. A crash in energy levels soon follows. As we try to restore that good feeling, we may indulge ourselves repeatedly, leading to an addictive cycle. In contrast, true self-care leads to more energy and natural good feelings that build over time. In addition, true self-care leads us to engage fully in life, rather than escape from it.

- **We believe self-care is too hard**—Some people neglect self-care because it seems too much like work or because they are afraid that they will fail.

- **We don't know any better**—We learn how to look after ourselves based on how well we were cared for when we were young. If our early caregivers neglected some area of our care, then as adults we may not know when we're neglecting ourselves, or that there is a better way to handle that area of our lives.

How Does Neglecting Self-Care Affect Our Energy?

When we neglect our self-care on any level of our being, we feel energetically drained. When we lack energy, it creates stress in many areas of our lives. The following describes what happens when we neglect our physical, emotional, mental or spiritual self-care.

The Effects of Neglecting Physical Self-Care

Proper physical care means providing ourselves with healthy amounts of nutritious food, water, exercise, sleep, fresh air, sunshine and relaxation.

When we neglect our physical self-care, we begin to feel tired. Every movement seems like a great effort. We feel sleepy and unable to concentrate. We have poor reflexes and our vision becomes poorer. So, we're more likely to have accidents on the road or at work. Our immunity weakens and we become more susceptible to illness.

We also find that it's much harder to stay positive emotionally and mentally, because our low physical vitality keeps dragging us down.

The Effects of Neglecting Emotional Self-Care

Proper emotional self-care means treating ourselves with love, compassion, forgiveness and respect. It also means allowing ourselves healthy emotional expression.

When we neglect emotional self-care, we may become depressed, weepy, irritable, angry, needy or clingy towards others, or else we may become emotionally numbed out. We may stop caring about others and become self-absorbed in our own troubles. We may also lash out at loved ones or co-workers for making demands on us, resulting in conflict and relationship difficulties.

The Effects of Neglecting Mental Self-Care

Proper mental self-care means feeding our minds with positive and life affirming thoughts. It means balancing work with play and setting proper boundaries on our time and responsibilities. It also involves stimulating our minds with opportunities to learn and grow.

When we neglect mental self-care through overwork, excessive responsibilities, self-judgment or perfectionism, we begin to feel burned out. This eventually leads to apathy, confusion and poor decisions. We lose our sense of perspective and feel more stressed by the events of life.

The Effects of Neglecting Spiritual Self-Care

Proper spiritual self-care means listening to our own heart and conscience. It also means that we allow ourselves to give and receive love, to enjoy beauty, to express our creativity, to follow our dreams and to contribute in some way to society.

When we neglect spiritual self-care, we may become pessimistic or negative, suspicious of the motives of others, disconnected from ourselves and alienated from others. We may feel unable to solve the problems in our lives and see our future as bleak and hopeless.

Or, we may feel angry and antisocial, seeing ourselves as victims of life's circumstances. And we may find ourselves making the same mistakes repeatedly without learning from them.

Neglecting One Type of Energy Affects the Others

Our physical, emotional, mental and spiritual energies interact. When we neglect self-care on one level, it also affects us on the others. For example, physical hunger can affect us emotionally (neediness), mentally (scarcity thinking), as well as spiritually (feeling helpless, abandoned by God or self).

However, this energetic interaction can also serve us, because when we begin to improve our self-care on any level of our energy field, the other levels will benefit as well. For example, when we improve our spiritual self-care by expressing creativity in a fun way, we find that our thinking becomes clearer, we feel happier emotionally and we feel physically more energized.

Why Make Self-Care a Top Priority?

We've all experienced the unpleasant effects of neglecting our self-care from time to time, especially when we're trying to cope with an emergency in our lives. We do our best to look after ourselves when the situation has passed, but inevitably, something else comes up and self-care again has to take a lower place in our priorities.

But what would happen if we made self-care non-optional? What if it stayed at the top of our list, no matter what happened? Is this something we could realistically achieve? And if so, how would that affect our lives?

Many of us equate self-care with having strict routines—a special diet, a workout program, visits to a therapist and so on. When we find our lives becoming too busy to keep up with the routine, we begin to feel bad about ourselves. We judge ourselves for not trying harder, for being unfit, undisciplined or lazy. When we criticize ourselves, it saps our energy even further. We then find it harder to motivate ourselves and may even give up trying.

So what does it take for us to make self-care a top priority? It takes the right mind-set: "I have value as a person and my energy levels are important for managing my life." With this attitude, we can make self-care a top priority and feel confident that it will provide us with the necessary energy to do everything else that is important to us.

The following describes what benefits we can expect when we make maintaining our physical, emotional, mental and spiritual energy a top priority in our lives:

The Benefits of More Physical Energy

Having plenty of physical energy gives us the confidence to try new or difficult things. It gives us more stamina and better balance, not only physically, but also emotionally. We're less easily thrown off or overwhelmed by the events in our lives.

Strong physical energy also strengthens our immune system and protects us from stress. And as our energy builds, we literally "glow with health" making us look and feel more attractive.

The Benefits of More Emotional Energy

When our emotional energy is strong and balanced, we feel a sense of inner joy that supports us regardless of what is happening in our lives. We become more openhearted and accepting towards others and ourselves. We no longer take things personally, but accept that others are simply behaving according to their own points of view. We listen and learn from each situation and then move on with our lives. We forgive the past and are at peace with ourselves.

The Benefits of More Mental Energy

When we feel mentally energized and balanced, we're better able to cope with both order and chaos. We become more open-minded, cheerful, optimistic, and have a greater sense of humor. And if a crisis arises, we're able to analyze our choices and arrive at a clear decision on what action to take. We also find ourselves better able to think of positive goals for ourselves and to plan the specific steps needed to achieve them.

The Benefits of More Spiritual Energy

When we feel spiritually more energized, we become confident and clear. We have a sense of purpose and meaning in our lives. We behave with generosity, integrity and honesty towards others and ourselves. Our creativity bubbles up and we enjoy exploring it in many ways. We also have a healthy curiosity about life. This helps us to learn and grow from all our experiences—from our failures as well as our successes. With each new life lesson, we develop our self-confidence and skills until eventually we're able to realize our dreams.

What Self-Care Do We Need for Better Energy?

Self-care is all about getting in touch with our real needs and then attending to them. And what we need varies from moment to moment and from situation to situation. That's why rigid self-care routines so often fall by the wayside, despite our best intentions. They simply do not support the reality that our lives and our needs are always changing.

So, the best approach to improving our energy is to connect frequently with ourselves and discover what we need in the present moment. It may take some time to learn how to listen to our own needs, but this will happen with practice.

How does such an approach work? Well, as our day progresses, we consider what our energy state is like in the moment and decide to change our energy as needed, exactly as Jane did in her Power Day in Chapter 1.

For example, the first thing Jane did when she woke up was to do a check-in of her energy on the physical, emotional, mental and spiritual levels. Realizing that her energies were low because of what happened the night before, she took the time to discover and attend to her needs.

Jane also took the time to be present with herself and do some breathing exercises (which you'll learn about in the next chapter) to strengthen herself just before her presentation to management. This gave her the clarity to deal with the questions after the talk and helped to bolster her self-confidence. Jane also made self-care decisions throughout the day that supported her energy levels.

As Jane's story shows us, by checking in with our energy regularly and making the necessary adjustments in our self-care, we can keep our energy strong and balanced throughout the day.

So, if you feel tired or low in energy, don't beat yourself up. Just do a check-in and see what you need to do for yourself in this moment.

What Do You Need Right Now?

The following exercise will help you to identify those areas where you need self-care and will help you to sense what actions you need to take to meet your needs right now.

Exercise 4-1: Self-Care Check-In

Have paper and pen handy to record notes.

1. Find a comfortable position and close your eyes.
2. Bring your attention to your breathing.

3. Take in a deep breath and let it out with a sigh. Repeat this 3 times.

4. Take another deep breath and allow your awareness to sink into your body.

5. Ask yourself the following questions:

    - Am I feeling any discomfort in my body right now? If so, where?
    - What is causing the discomfort?
    - What does that part of my body need from me to feel better?
    - What is one thing, however small, that I can do right now to help meet this need?

6. Take another deep breath and allow your awareness to move into your emotional energy.

7. Ask yourself the following questions:

    - Am I feeling any emotional discomfort right now? If so, what emotion is calling for my attention?
    - What does this emotion need from me right now to feel better?
    - What is one thing, however small, that I can do right now to help meet this need?

8. Take another deep breath and allow your awareness to move into your mental energy.

9. Ask yourself the following questions:
   - Am I feeling any mental discomfort right now? If so, what thoughts are calling for my attention?
   - What does my mind need right now to feel clearer?
   - What is one thing, however small, that I can do right now to help meet this need?
10. Take another deep breath and allow your awareness to move into your spiritual energy.
11. Ask yourself the following questions:
    - Am I feeling any spiritual discomfort right now? If so, what is my heart or conscience telling me about this right now?
    - What do I need to help me feel better about my life or myself?
    - What is one thing, however small, that I can do right now to help meet this need?
12. When you're finished, take another deep breath and let it out with a sigh.
13. Open your eyes and make a note of your experiences.

When you commit to making self-care a top priority, you'll become alert to what you need and over time, you'll discover new ways of meeting those needs.

For example, when you do a check-in for your physical energy, you might sense your body wants more movement—that your life has become too sedentary. Being aware of that need puts your subconscious on the alert for a way to solve the problem. Fifteen minutes later, you're chatting with a friend and they casually mention they want to go cycling. You suddenly think, "Hey, I could do that!"

You try it and feel great afterwards—this is your body's way of telling you that a need was met. You find yourself wanting to do it again and soon cycling becomes a regular part of your life. What's important is that you do it, not because you "should" exercise, but because you have fun doing it and it feels physically rewarding.

Or you might have the opposite problem: your life is so busy you're constantly on the go. When you do a check-in, you might become aware of a deep tiredness and a need to simply rest and do nothing. Your subconscious mind will again look for ways to help you meet that need. Later, you see a flyer for a new day spa near you that's offering an opening special. Because you're alert to your need, the flyer grabs your attention. Suddenly it feels right to do this and even though you're busy, you book a two-hour package at the spa. You go after work and later emerge from the session feeling relaxed and refreshed. You've met your need for rest and rejuvenation in that moment.

When we regularly check in with ourselves and fine-tune our self-care to meet our needs in the moment, the result is more energy, a happier mood, a clearer mind and a positive more creative outlook on life. When we make self-care a top priority in our lives, it is easy to see how we can transform every day into a Power Day, just as Jane did in Chapter 1.

Summary

Anytime we feel discomfort physically, emotionally, mentally or spiritually, it means that we need self-care. When we learn to pay attention to our needs and take proper action in the moment, we soon discover we have more energy in our lives for the people and activities that are important to us.

With practice and experimentation, we discover that taking proper care of ourselves doesn't need to take much time. Many self-care actions take just a few minutes and yet greatly improve our energy. The next chapter introduces several excellent techniques for managing our energy throughout the day and for coping with specific situations. These are quick exercises, so you'll find it easy to fit them into even a busy day and be able to boost your energy when you need it most.

CHAPTER 5

Maintaining Your Energy

As we've seen in the previous chapters, our energy levels strongly affect how well we're able to function in our lives. So you might wonder if there's anything we can do to build and maintain a healthy level of energy. There is—provided you understand how energy works.

There are four basic laws governing energy:

- **Energy flows from high to low**—Like water flowing downhill, energy flows from high to low. That is, energy will flow from a source of high energy to a source of lower energy. This explains why if you're around someone who is ill, you may start to feel drained as your energy automatically flows towards them to fill their field.

- **Like energies attract**—We tend to feel comfortable with people who have similar energy to us. People are attracted to like-minded people. Similarly, one negative thought will evoke more of the same from other people.

- **Energy follows thought**—Thoughts are a form of energy and have an influence on other types of energy. When we judge ourselves negatively, it affects the rest of our energy and we begin to feel physically tired.

   However, we can instead make use of this law to improve our energy state, by consciously holding loving and encouraging thoughts toward ourselves. This is how creative visualization works to bring about healing or reduce stress. It's also the principle that explains the healing power of prayer, even at a distance.

- **Energy moves in cycles**—Like everything else in nature, our energy is affected by the seasons, times of day, cycles of light and dark, as well as temperature cycles. Like the moon and the tides, our energy expands and contracts in phases.

   When our energy is expanding and increasing, we feel wonderful, on top of the world and ready to tackle anything. Inevitably, however, our energy comes to the end of the expansion phase and begins to contract.

   During the contraction phase, our energy moves inward to recharge. We typically feel quiet, tired or unfocussed in this phase. After recharging, our energy naturally begins a new expansion.

We can make use of these four energy laws to build and strengthen our energy levels. Like following an exercise program at the gym, it takes regular and consistent practice to build our energy. We also need to be able to maintain our energy levels to keep ourselves from being depleted by the stresses that we face during our day.

The most important tools for building and maintaining our energy are:

- **Conscious breathing**—Breathing mindfully to reduce stress and to improve brain function
- **Grounding**—Connecting to the earth's energy field for more stability, endurance and strength
- **Charging**—Boosting your energy levels as needed
- **Clearing**—Getting rid of unwanted energies from your field or environment

This chapter describes each of these energy tools in detail and provides step-by-step instructions for using these skills to strengthen your own energy.

Conscious Breathing

How we breathe has a strong effect on the body. When threatened, many people hold their breath or only take shallow breaths. Both reactions reduce the amount of oxygen available to the brain.

Inadequate oxygen stresses the body and creates anxiety. Without enough oxygen to the brain, we can't think straight to deal with a potential threat. So, our breath is truly important.

Our breathing reactions happen so automatically that most of us don't even notice them. However, unlike many other systems in the body, our breath is under our conscious control. We can change how we breathe any time we want. We do this when we hold our breath while swimming underwater, for example.

Conscious breathing is probably the most fundamental tool that we have for managing our energy. Simply slowing our breathing and focusing our awareness on the flow of our breath helps to calm us. It makes us aware of the present moment. Physiologically, the added oxygen nourishes the brain, reduces anxiety and provides more mental clarity for resolving the situation.

Conscious breathing is the quickest way to change your energy. So let's look at some exercises to bring mindfulness to the breath and see how this affects our energy.

The Complete Breath

Most people breathe incompletely even under normal conditions because of poor posture (slouching or slumping). They typically use only their upper part of their lungs. A proper complete breath, however, makes use of the whole lung capacity. The following exercise will help you to experience the benefits of full breathing.

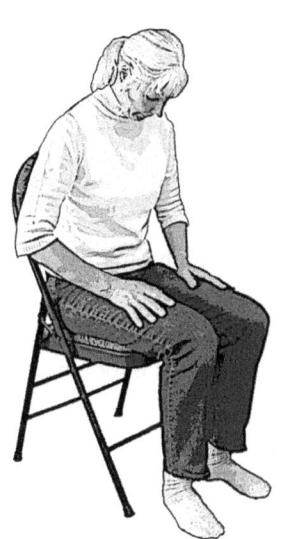 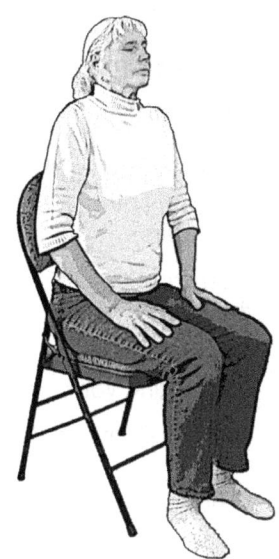

Exercise 5-1: The Complete Breath

Exercise 5-1: The Complete Breath

Have paper and pen handy to record notes.

1. Sit in a comfortable position.

2. Perform the Complete Breath as follows:

   - Breathe out through the mouth, contracting your stomach to empty your lungs completely.

   - Immediately, begin to inhale through the nose. As you breathe in, slowly expand your belly to fill the lower part of the lungs.

- Continuing to inhale, expand your chest to fill the middle part of your lungs.
- Still inhaling, raise your shoulders to fill the upper part of your lungs until you can't breathe in any more air.
- Now, breathe out through the nose. As you slowly breathe out, empty the upper part of your lungs first by lowering the shoulders.
- Then continue to breathe out and empty the middle part of the lungs by collapsing the chest.
- Still breathing out, empty the bottom part of the lungs by contracting your abdomen until all the air is expelled.

3. Perform the Complete Breath five times.
4. Relax and breathe normally, paying attention to how your body feels.
5. Record your experience in your notes.

The Calming Breath

While the Complete Breath will help to reduce anxiety in any situation, the Calming Breath will retrain your body to hold a calm state most of the time. With practice, this exercise gradually increases your lung capacity so you have more oxygen available to you in your daily life. Then, when a crisis occurs, you're not looking for your breath or hyperventilating, because you already have a plentiful reserve of oxygen to deal with whatever is going on.

Exercise 5-2: The Calming Breath

Have paper and pen handy to record notes.

1. Sit in a comfortable position.
2. Breathe out through the mouth, contracting your stomach to empty your lungs completely.
3. Perform the Calming Breath as follows:
   - Breathe in through your nose for a slow count of four, making sure to fill your lungs completely as described in Exercise 5-1.
   - Hold your breath in for a slow count of four.
   - Now, breathe out through your nose for a slow count of four, making sure to empty your lungs completely.
   - Hold your out-breath for a slow count of four.
4. Repeat the Calming Breath five times.
5. Relax and breathe normally, paying attention to how your body feels.
6. Record your experience in your notes.

The Cleansing Breath

The Cleansing Breath helps your lungs to oxygenate your blood more efficiently and helps to move toxins out of your system.

Exercise 5-3: The Cleansing Breath

Have paper and pen handy to record notes.

1. Sit in a comfortable position.
2. Breathe out through the mouth, contracting your stomach to empty your lungs completely.
3. Perform the Cleansing Breath as follows:
   - Breathe in through your nose for a slow count of four, making sure to fill your lungs completely, as described in Exercise 5-1.
   - Hold your breath in for a slow count of eight.
   - Now, breathe out through your nose for a slow count of four, making sure to empty your lungs completely.
   - Hold your out-breath for a slow count of eight.
4. Repeat the Cleansing Breath five times.
5. Relax and breathe normally, paying attention to how your body feels.
6. Record your experience in your notes.

Combining Breathing with Visualization

When we learn to combine conscious breathing with visualization, we can use the breath to calm ourselves in a crisis. We can also use it in physical emergencies to speed healing. When we hurt ourselves, if we start breathing deeply while visualizing health, we'll heal much more quickly.

Claudette describes how she used this technique as a form of energy first aid:

"I wanted to remove the pit from an avocado. I was using one of the sharpest kitchen knives, and although my mother had warned me many times "Do not stab the pit of an avocado," I did it anyway. Sure enough, the knife slipped and I stabbed myself right in the fleshy part of my hand! It was so painful. I saw all the blood and immediately I thought of stitches and hospitals.

"Then I thought, 'No. Don't put your energy there. Put your energy in healing.' So, I brought the skin together and started breathing deeply. I pictured my hand as whole and healthy, using my other hand as a reminder of what that looked like. As I breathed, I became more in touch with the healing that was going on. By the end of the day, the skin had mended. I didn't even need a bandage!"

Because energy follows thought, when we combine conscious breathing with visualization we're moving energy. We can use this technique to change our energy in the physical, emotional, mental or spiritual parts of our being.

For instance, when we visualize breathing out stress and breathing in calmness, we create a state of inner peace and presence that enables us to deal more effectively with stressful situations.

We can also use visualization with the breath to clear and change our emotional states. Claudette uses this technique whenever she goes to the dentist:

> *"When I was a child, I was terrified of going to the dentist. So while sitting in the dentist's chair, I would focus all my attention on my breathing and imagine being in a warm sunny place. And I wouldn't notice the dentist was working on my teeth. I didn't even feel the needle going in, and in those days, they used big needles! I still use this technique today whenever I go to the dentist."*

On the mental level, if our minds are too busy and our thoughts running over the same scenarios again and again, then we can picture breathing out the circling thoughts and breathing in clarity instead.

When we're worried about something, we can focus on our breathing and visualize the outcome that we would like, rather than the outcome that we fear. We'll find that our minds become much more productive and solutions to the problem will come to us more easily.

Because our energies affect other people, when we worry about others, we place an energetic burden on them. It's far better to breathe out the worry and breathe in what we want for them instead—for example joy, happiness, success or health. That changes the focus of the energy and actually helps them to achieve those positive experiences instead.

The following exercise will give you an experience of combining conscious breathing with visualization.

Exercise 5-4: Combining Breathing with Visualization

Have paper and pen handy to record notes.

1. Sit in a comfortable position.
2. Perform the Complete Breath as described in Exercise 5-1.
3. As you inhale, visualize that you're breathing in life force into every cell of your body. As you breathe out, visualize that you're breathing out stress from every cell of your body.
4. Repeat the exercise four or five times. Then relax and breathe normally, paying attention to how your body feels afterwards.
5. Record your experience in your notes.

Try practicing this exercise using different visualizations, for example:

- **Joy**—As you inhale, imagine that you're breathing joy into your field. As you exhale, imagine that you're releasing any stressful emotions from your field, such as anxiety or anger.

- **Gratitude**—As you inhale, imagine that you're breathing gratitude into your field. As you exhale, imagine that you're releasing any negative or stressful thoughts from your field, such as judgment or perfectionism.

- **Success**—As you inhale, imagine that you're breathing success into your life. As you exhale, imagine that you're releasing failure from your life.

You can make up your own visualization—simply imagine breathing in whatever you want to have more of in your life and breathing out whatever you want to release from your life. You can also play with this technique while doing physical exercise. For example, while running, you can breathe in more energy and breathe out fatigue. Or, you could breathe in the future you want, imagining it coming toward you as you run, and breathe out the past, imagining it falling away behind you. While practicing yoga, you can breathe in relaxation and release stiffness as you breathe out.

Other Breathing Techniques

Conscious breathing techniques have been studied and perfected in India and other ancient cultures for thousands of years. Because many of these techniques can have a powerful effect on your body and on your energy, it's important to practice them under the supervision of a qualified instructor. Most schools of yoga offer such training.

Grounding
(Connecting to the Earth)

"Grounding" is the act of connecting and synchronizing your own energy field with the earth's energy field. Just as our physical bodies need food, water, sunlight and air to function optimally, our energy bodies need to take in energy from the earth. When we disconnect from the earth, it's as though we're running on batteries. And as everyone knows, batteries eventually run down.

Grounding happens naturally when we're relaxed and fully present in our bodies. However, in our culture most of us spend our lives in our heads, feeling anything but relaxed. To complicate matters, we're often also sleep-deprived, overworked, overstimulated (for example, by TV, movies, music, video games, drugs, caffeine) and completely out of touch with our natural rhythms.

Then we begin to depend on artificial substitutes to boost our energy—energy bars, energy shakes, coffee, drugs, even "runner's high". But these substitutes have side effects. They only provide a temporary energy boost, typically followed by a crash.

However, when we know how to ground, we don't have to run on "batteries." We can instead plug directly into the earth's energy field, at any time, to access the energy we need for health.

Being grounded helps to:

- Boost our energy
- Stabilize and calm our emotions (particularly when combined with deep breathing)
- Give us a sense of connection with all of life
- Heighten our energy senses
- Become present in our bodies
- Strengthen our energy fields

Staying grounded while engaging in sports or other strenuous activities keeps our energy strong so we can go farther—it gives us endurance. This is a great skill for runners, hikers, golfers and other athletes. Grounding also increases our ability to tolerate pain.

The Effects of Being Ungrounded

What happens when we're not grounded? Typical symptoms include:

- Feeling scattered and easily distracted
- Forgetfulness or absentmindedness
- Neediness
- Low vitality
- Being easily upset or unbalanced by others

- Clumsiness

- Feeling overwhelmed or overstimulated

- Feeling isolated, confused or lost (unable to find your bearings)

How to Ground

This section will show you how to ground and will provide some exercises to give you a direct experience of what earth energy feels like and what you can do with it.

Basic Grounding Technique

Exercise 5-5 describes the basic technique for grounding.

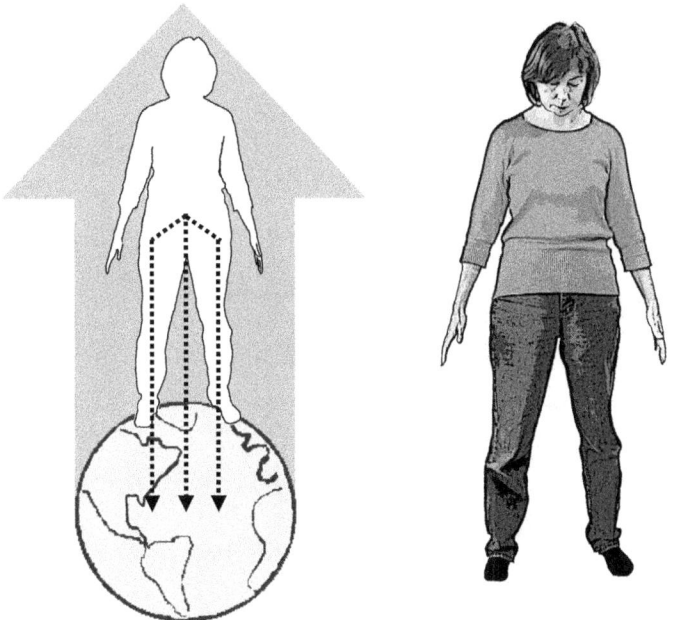

Exercise 5-5: Grounding to the Earth

Exercise 5-5: Grounding

Have paper and pen handy to record notes.

1. Stand with your feet comfortably apart and knees slightly bent.
2. Perform the Complete Breath a few times (see *Exercise 5-1: The Complete Breath* on page 93).
3. Visualize sending energy roots down your spine and down both legs deep into the earth. Keep sending the roots deeper until you feel them "click" into the center of the earth.
4. Continue breathing deeply and notice what happens to your energy.
5. Now, let go of your connection to the earth. How does that feel?
6. Repeat the exercise a few times, asking yourself the following questions:
    - How does breathing affect my energy?
    - How does grounding affect my energy?
    - How does lack of grounding affect my energy?
7. Record your experience in your notes.

Grounding with a Partner

Try the following exercise with a friend:

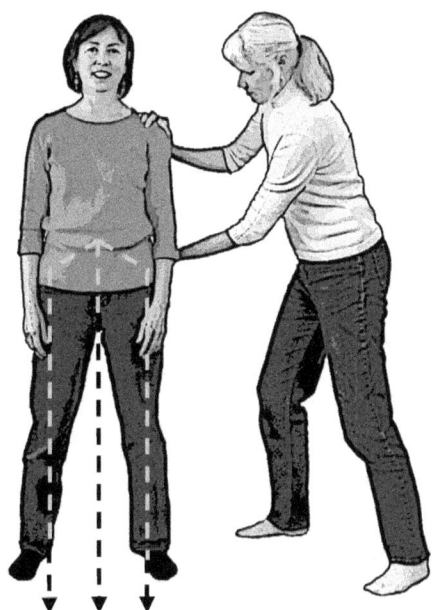

Exercise 5-6: Grounding with a Partner

Exercise 5-6: Grounding Exercises with a Partner

Have paper and pen handy to record notes.

1. Stand with your feet comfortably apart and knees slightly bent.

2. Ask your partner to try to push you or pull you off balance. What happens?

3. Now ground (see *Exercise 5-5: Grounding* on page 104) and while staying grounded, ask your partner to try it again. Is it easier or harder for you to keep your balance when grounded?

> 4. Try to push or pull your partner off balance while they are ungrounded and then again while they're grounded. What happens?
> 5. Record your experience in your notes.

Other Things to Try

Practice your grounding in different life situations and notice how being grounded or ungrounded affects you. Here are some things to explore:

- **Endurance**—Try walking up a long hill with and without grounding.

- **Pain tolerance**—The next time you feel pain, try grounding and see if you feel better or worse.

- **Sense of confidence**—In a situation where you feel nervous, like public speaking, try grounding and see how that affects you.

- **Emotional stability**—If you find yourself upset with someone, try grounding and see what happens.

- **Mental clarity**—The next time you feel stumped or overwhelmed by a problem, try grounding and see how that affects you.

- **Intuitive awareness**—If you need to make an important decision, try grounding first and see what happens.

When to Ground

Grounding is helpful in many life situations. Here are some examples:

- **On the telephone**—When we want to end a conversation, but keep getting dragged further into the other person's story, it helps to ground and to hold our energy within our bubble. We don't even have to say anything. This keeps us from feeding their story with our energy. The other person eventually will stop talking. At that moment, we become able to say, "I have to go now."

  An even better solution is to begin grounding before answering the phone. When we remember to do this, we can usually prevent the situation from occurring in the first place.

- **Making a complaint**—If we're making a complaint about something that matters to us, sometimes it happens that the other person insists on justifying their position without considering our point of view. We may feel frustrated, angry and powerless. Our emotional state can distort our perception of the situation. The next thing we know, we start arguing with the other person. Unfortunately, instead of resolving the problem, this only makes things worse and we lose whatever potential cooperation may have existed in the other person.

  Grounding, however, gives us a reality check. It brings us quickly back into our bodies and energy fields. From there it's easy to remember to put our bubble back into place. When we're grounded and in the safety of our bubble, we immediately realize that fighting isn't going to get us anywhere and so instead, we begin to focus on finding a solution.

Grounding allows this whole sequence to take place in a few moments. We're able to "hold our ground" on this important issue, while making our point in such a way that the other person is finally able to hear us.

Note that holding our ground does not mean walking over someone else. On the contrary, when we know how to ground, we're able to make allowances for others and even help them. If they are emotionally reacting to the situation, we can ground first and strengthen our bubble. This calms us and helps calm them, too.

We can use our clarity and composure to bring everyone involved back to what is really happening. This gives us a better chance of gaining their cooperation to arrive at a win-win solution.

- **At airports**—It is easy to feel distracted at airports because so much is going on around us—signs, people, sounds, lights, voices, food, fear of flying, public announcements and security—all of these things overwhelm our senses. Our thoughts are all over the place and it's hard to stay focused. We feel "scattered".

Grounding can help us to anchor ourselves and to become present. Then we can use the energy bubble to create safety so we can relax and enjoy our trip.

- **Medical emergencies**—Grounding helps to reduce anxiety and bring our energies back into our bodies so we can deal with what is happening in the moment. It's a quick way to bring us out of panic and back into a practical state of mind. It also provides the body with extra energy and strength to cope with healing.

  Grounding can also help protect us from the onset of shock. Gail shares the following experience of using grounding in a medical emergency:

  "A few of years ago, my father tripped and fell, injuring his eye badly. I instinctively grounded and immediately felt calmness and strength flood my body. I knelt behind him on the pavement and held my arms around him, with one hand protecting his eye. Holding him while I grounded automatically caused his energy to ground, too. In effect, I was grounding for both of us. This helped to protect him from shock and kept me calm enough to deal with the situation. My father also managed to stay calm and clear for over 12 hours while he waited in the hospital for emergency surgery."

- **Dangerous situations**—Danger can cause us to react in panic or terror, which can have fatal results. Grounding helps us to feel stable, strong and present enough to be able to put our bubble back in place, so we can think clearly to deal with the danger. Claudette relates this experience:

"Many years ago, I worked in a place that helped people with mental illness to learn how to cope in society. The facility provided 24-hour support and sometimes I worked the night shift, staying overnight. In the middle of the night, one of the patients came into my room holding a large kitchen knife. "I don't want to do this, but I have to kill you," she said.

"I immediately grounded and sent up a prayer. I had been working closely with her and I knew that she heard voices in her head that would tell her to do strange things. I needed to be very cautious. "Oh yes?" I said, trying to sound calm. I then began a conversation with her to elicit her cooperation. It took a long time. And I continued to ground and pray the whole time, because I had to be so present not only for her, but also for myself. Eventually I was able to take the knife from her without harm."

- **Driving in poor conditions**—When we drive in difficult conditions, such as in snow or ice, it takes all of our concentration to make it safely to our destination. Our normal driving reflexes don't work in these conditions, so we have to pay more attention to what is happening in the moment. A slip of our attention can cause an accident.

Grounding helps us to stay calm and present. It also provides added mental clarity to respond to the situation. Gail shares her experience of using grounding while driving:

"When it snows in Vancouver, it causes a traffic nightmare. Most residents are not used to driving in snow conditions and accidents abound. One morning there was 30 cm (about 12 inches) of freshly fallen snow on the ground, and I had to go to a doctor's

appointment. As I got in the car, I took a deep breath and grounded. Before driving off, I consciously visualized a safe, easy, quick and enjoyable journey.

"Grounding while driving kept me present and open to intuitive information. I felt no fear. I simply noticed how the snow was affecting my ability to steer and brake and adjusted my driving to compensate for it. As I neared my destination, I intuitively sensed I should use a side road to approach the building, rather than my usual route via the main street.

"When I got to my doctor's office, I learned the main street in front of the building was inaccessible because of a major accident. People around me were swearing about the weather and the traffic delays, some had accidents and many people were having a bad day because of the snow. I, on the other hand, had a different day—peaceful, calm and even enjoyable. Grounding works!"

Charging

Grounding by itself will automatically start charging our fields, but just like a battery, if our energy is already low, it will take some time to recharge us to normal. However, when we combine conscious breathing and visualization with grounding, we can charge our energy fields quickly anytime we need to—these skills combine to turbo-boost our energy.

How to Charge Your Energy Field

In this section, you'll learn some techniques for boosting your energy quickly. We recommend that you do a check-in before and after each exercise to discover for yourself how each exercise affects you.

Basic Charging Technique

The following exercise will give a strong boost to your physical energies. This exercise is a good one to do when you need extra strength before some physically demanding task.

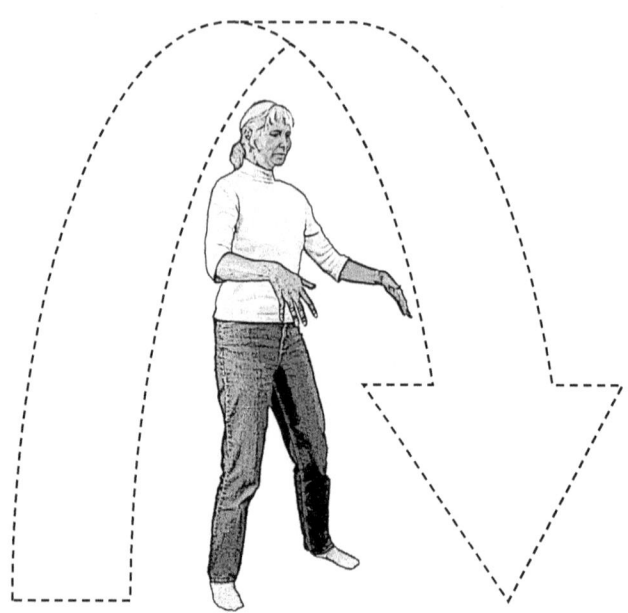

Exercise: 5-7: Basic Charging Technique

> ### *Exercise 5-7: Basic Charging Technique*
>
> Have paper and pen handy to record notes.
>
> 1. Stand with your feet comfortably apart and knees slightly bent.
> 2. Ground yourself to the earth. (See *Exercise 5-5: Grounding* on page 104.)
> 3. Breathe deeply while visualizing as follows:
>   - As you inhale, imagine drawing energy up from the earth through your grounding roots, into your feet, into your legs, up your spine and into your chest and arms.
>   - As you breathe out, imagine directing the energy with your hands into your energy field.
> 4. Repeat ten times or until you feel energized.
> 5. Record your experience in your notes.

Charging with Different Energy Frequencies

The next exercise helps to charge your energy field on physical, emotional, mental and spiritual parts of your being, using various color frequencies of energy. Each color has a unique healing and energizing effect on the body and energy field.

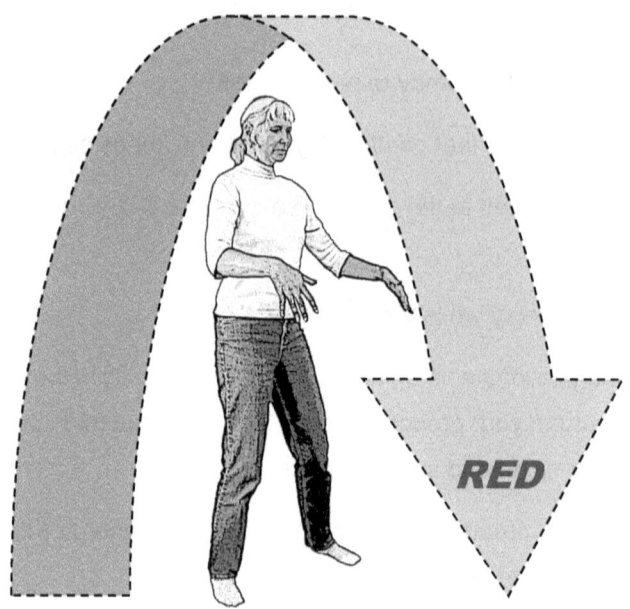

Exercise 5-8: Color Breathing Exercise

As you do the exercise, try to sense how each color frequency affects your body, your emotions, your mind and your spirit differently.

Exercise 5-8: Color Breathing Exercise

Have paper and pen handy to record notes.

1. Stand with your feet comfortably apart and knees slightly bent.
2. Ground yourself to the earth. (See *Exercise 5-5: Grounding* on page 104.)

3. Breathe deeply while visualizing as follows:

   - Breathe in the color *bright red* (like ripe strawberries) up from the earth. Then breathe that color out into your energy field.
   - Repeat until your energy field is full of bright red energy.
   - Pause to notice how this red energy affects your body, your emotions, your thoughts and your spirit.

4. Now, breathe deeply while visualizing as follows:

   - Breathe in the color *reddish orange* (like a tangerine) up from the earth. Then breathe that color out into your energy field.
   - Repeat until your energy field is full of this orange energy.
   - Pause to notice how this orange energy affects your body, your emotions, your thoughts and your spirit.

5. Now, breathe deeply while visualizing as follows:

   - Breathe in the color *bright yellow* (like a lemon) up from the earth. Then breathe that color out into your energy field.
   - Repeat until your energy field is full of bright yellow energy.
   - Pause to notice how this yellow energy affects your body, your emotions, your thoughts and your spirit.

6. Now, breathe deeply while visualizing as follows:

   - Breathe in the color *green* (like new grass) up from the earth. Then breathe that color out into your energy field.
   - Repeat until your energy field is full of green energy.
   - Pause to notice how this green energy affects your body, your emotions, your thoughts and your spirit.

7. Now, breathe deeply while visualizing as follows:
   - Breathe in the color *bright blue* (like a summer sky) up from the earth. Then breathe out that color into your energy field.
   - Repeat until your energy field is full of bright blue energy.
   - Pause to notice how this blue energy affects your body, your emotions, your thoughts and your spirit.
8. Now, breathe deeply while visualizing as follows:
   - Breathe in the color *indigo* (dark inky blue—like the midnight sky) from the earth. Then breathe that color out into your energy field.
   - Repeat until your energy field is full of indigo energy.
   - Pause to notice how this indigo energy affects your body, your emotions, your thoughts and your spirit.
9. Now, breathe deeply while visualizing as follows:
   - Breathe in the color *brilliant white* (like starlight) up from the earth. Then breathe out that color into your energy field.
   - Repeat until your energy field is full of sparkling white energy.
   - Pause to notice how this color of energy affects your body, your emotions, your thoughts and your spirit.
10. Record your experience in your notes.

Other Things to Try

You can also do the color breathing exercise while moving around to music. As you experience the color, imagine what music might provide the same frequency. Many people find native drumming resonates with the red energy, while Middle Eastern music or jazz saxophone resonates with the orange energy.

You can also experiment with different types of movement to match the color frequencies. For example, the red energy might inspire a marching or stamping dance, where your feet make strong, flat contact with the earth. The orange energy might inspire movements that are more sensuous or even a belly dance!

With practice, you'll become familiar with how each of the different color frequencies affects you. Then you can begin to charge your field with specific colors to suit any situation. For example, if you need an emotional boost, you might try breathing in orange and dancing to some sensual music. If you need mental clarity, you could charge your field with yellow energy, while listening to some Baroque music, like Bach or Vivaldi. Have fun with it and explore what works best for you.

When to Charge Your Energy

Ideally, we should charge our fields every day, preferably first thing in the morning. It's best to avoid charging our energy at night before bed. We may find it hard to get to sleep—like too much caffeine! However, if we need to work a night shift, then charging our energy before leaving for work helps to keep us refreshed and awake for our night duties.

Other instances where it helps to charge our energy include:

- **When we need to stay awake**—operating machinery, night driving or dealing with jet lag
- **When we feel depleted**—after visiting a sick relative or listening to a long boring conversation
- **When we're unable to concentrate**—feeling sleepy at work after a heavy lunch
- **When we need an extra boost of physical energy**—before a race or before doing something physically challenging, like working out
- **When we feel cold or hungry**—to help keep us going until warmth or food is available

And there are many other occasions where charging is useful—experiment to find out what works for you!

Clearing Unwanted Energies

If you did the exercises earlier in this book, by now you've experienced how the energy of places, groups and objects can affect us positively or negatively. When your energy awareness becomes more sensitive, you may start to notice that unwanted energies have collected in your field.

For example:

- You visit a sick friend in hospital. When you come home, you notice that you still feel the tense atmosphere of the hospital affecting you.
- A coworker snaps at you and you feel irritable for the rest of the day.
- After watching the nightly news or a violent movie on TV, you feel fearful and pessimistic about life.
- You spent an hour deleting hundreds of spam e-mail messages and you feel "sticky" afterwards.

Just as you wash off the dust after working outside, so you can wash off the "psychic dust" that you pick up during your day.

How to Clear Your Energy Field

Because energy follows thought, an excellent way to clear your energy field is to use visualization, especially when you combine it with the breath and movement. Here are some techniques for clearing your field of unwanted energies.

Note: As you perform each exercise, stay fully present in the body and sense what is happening to your energy. This will give you a direct experience of what clearing feels like energetically.

The Waterfall Cleanse

Do the following exercise daily. When finished, you'll have a feeling of lightness and relaxation.

A great time to do the Waterfall Cleanse technique is while taking a shower—you just imagine sending the psychic dirt down the drain.

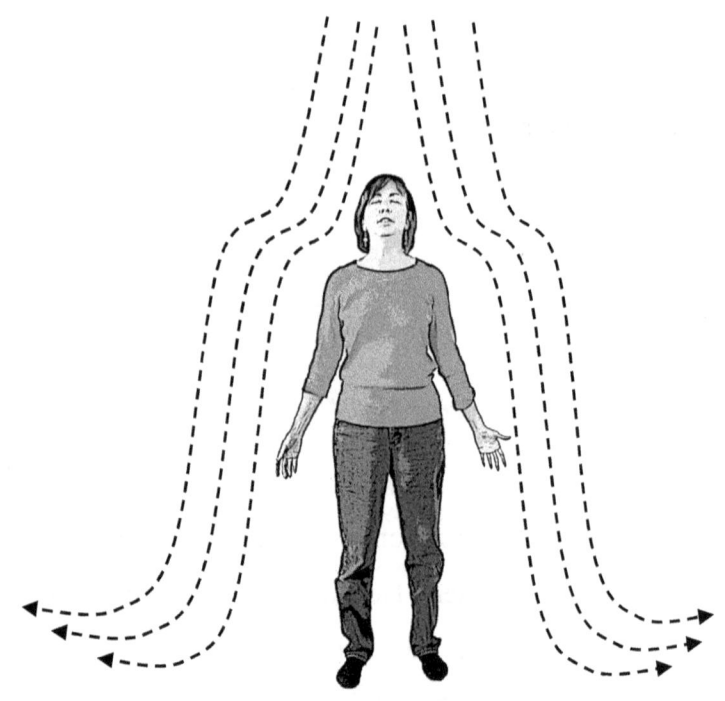

Exercise 5-9: The Waterfall Cleanse

Exercise 5-9: Waterfall Cleanse

Have paper and pen handy to record notes.

1. Stand with your feet comfortably apart and knees slightly bent.
2. Ground yourself to the earth. (See *Exercise 5-5: Grounding* on page 104.)
3. Imagine yourself standing under a waterfall with a river at your feet leading outside.

   - Feel the water splash over your head, your shoulders, your chest and back down your legs.
   - Feel the waterfall wash away all the old emotions and distracting thoughts that have gathered about you during the day.
   - Imagine the water pouring into the river and carrying the unwanted energy away. Perform this exercise slowly, giving careful attention to each part of your body.

4. Repeat the whole exercise once more.
5. Record your experience in your notes.

Aura Brushing

You can do this next exercise, Aura Brushing, by itself or together with the Waterfall Cleanse.

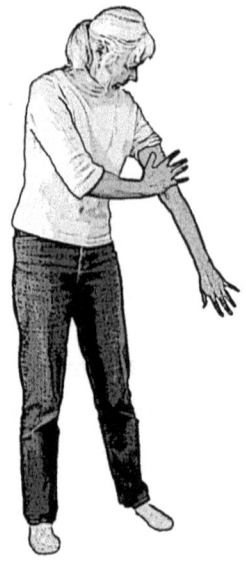

Exercise 5-10: Aura Brushing

Exercise 5-10: Aura Brushing

Have paper and pen handy to record notes.

1. Stand with your feet comfortably apart and knees slightly bent.
2. Ground yourself to the earth. (See *Exercise 5-5: Grounding* on page 104.)
3. Gently brush your fingers about an inch above the skin down your body and limbs, as if you're brushing off dust.

> 4. While brushing, imagine that your hands are removing the thick layer of old energy. Be aware of the sensation in your palms and fingers as the energy that you're brushing off builds up on your hands.
> 5. Flick the collected energy off your hands as you brush.
> 6. Repeat the whole exercise a few times until you feel lighter and cleaner.
> 7. Follow up with a brief charging exercise to fill your field with positive energy (see *Exercise 5-7: Basic Charging Technique* on page 113).
> 8. Record your experience in your notes.

Aura Brushing with a Partner

The Aura Brushing exercise is also fun to do with a partner or a group of friends. If doing this exercise in a group, stand in a circle facing one another. Then have each person take a turn being in the center of the circle, while the rest of the group cleans that person's field.

When it's your turn to receive the Aura Brushing, simply stand in a grounded position and stay present in your body, noticing the energies move as your partner or friends clear your field.

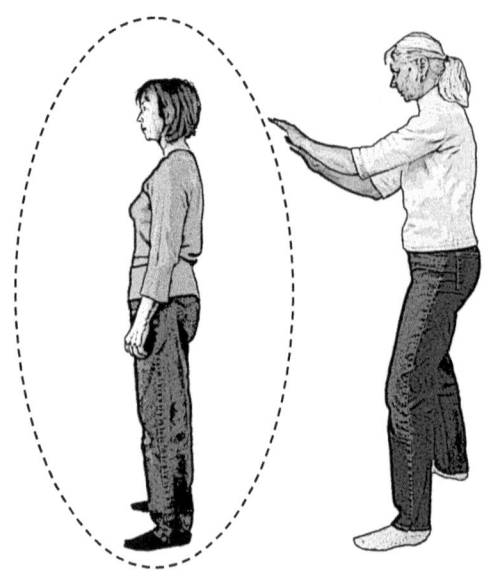

Figure 5-11: Aura Brushing with a Partner

Exercise 5-11: Aura Brushing with a Partner or Group

Have paper and pen handy to record notes.

The partner or group members giving the Aura Brushing should perform the following steps:

1. Stand with your feet comfortably apart and knees slightly bent, facing the person who is receiving the Aura Brushing.

2. Ground yourself to the earth. (See *Exercise 5-5: Grounding* on page 104.)

3. Starting at the head, gently sweep your fingers a few inches above the skin down the receiving person's aura, as if you're brushing off dust.

4. While brushing, imagine that your hands are removing the thick layer of old energy. Be aware of the sensation in your palms and fingers as the energy that you're brushing off builds up on your hands. Make long strokes from the head down to the feet.

5. After you reach the feet, put your hands on the ground to send the collected energy off your hands into the earth.

6. Step to another side of the person and repeat the whole exercise again. Continue to work around the person until you return to your starting position. If you're in a circle, the whole circle rotates until everyone has returned to their starting position, while the person in the middle stays still.

7. Do a brief charging exercise to fill your field with positive energy (see *Exercise 5-7: Basic Charging Technique* on page 113). Then direct the energy through your fingers into the person's field, imagining that you're "fluffing out" their field with positive energy.

8. Change positions and repeat the exercise until each partner or group member has had a turn at receiving.

9. Record your experiences in your notes. Then share your perceptions with your partner or other group members.

How to Clear Your Environment

When our living space feels energetically contaminated by negative or foreign energy, it feels unsafe to us. It no longer feels like "home". For example, when people discover that their house has been burgled, they typically feel violated. They can subconsciously sense traces of the burglar's energy imprinted in the walls and furnishings of their home.

Some other experiences that can energetically contaminate our environment include arguments, violence, general abuse, chronic illness, depression, grief and neglect.

Fortunately, just as we can clear our own energy fields of unwanted energy, it's an easy matter to cleanse our home and return it to a state of calm and safety. Here's a simple technique that works well:

Exercise 5-12: Clearing Environmental Energies

Have paper and pen handy to record notes.

1. Open all the doors and windows and allow fresh air to circulate in the room for at least 15 minutes.
2. During this time, ground into the earth (see *Exercise 5-5: Grounding* on page 104) and do one of the following:

    - Imagine sunshine filling the area and dissolving all unwanted energies.
    - Light incense or a bundle of dried sage and fan the smoke around the room.
    - Combine ten drops of lavender essential oil with two cups of warm water in a spray bottle, shake it up and spray throughout the space.
    - Imagine a pristine forest or waterfall in each room.
    - Laugh, clap, sing, drum or dance enthusiastically with family members around the room.

3. The room should feel pleasant and clean after this. If not, try some of the other suggestions in step 2 until the space feels good to you.
4. Repeat steps 1 through 3 for each room that holds negative energy.
5. After clearing the environment, reclaim your space by going into your energy bubble and expanding your loving energy to fill your entire home. Invite other members of your family to do the same, especially with their own rooms.
6. Record your experience in your notes.

When to Clear Unwanted Energies

When we've developed our energy awareness, we intuitively know when we need to clear our fields or our environment—the energy feels "sticky." It's a bit like how we feel when we get sweaty or dirty.

A good rule of thumb is to clear our fields anytime we've experienced something negative, such as:

- Illness (our own or someone else's)
- A lot of heavy emotional energy from someone else (such as anger or grief)
- Witnessing verbal or physical violence
- Any situation that depresses us or makes us uncomfortable

Similarly, we should clear our living space when such negative experiences happen inside the home.

Note: It's a good habit to create an energy bubble around our homes whenever we enter or leave them. The positive energy tends to discourage intruders and helps to create a loving environment in which to live.

Daily Energy Maintenance

You now have a variety of techniques at your disposal that you can use to strengthen and maintain your energy. Begin to practice them often so they become reliable tools that are easy for you to remember. The best way to do this is to start to integrate them into your day. The following is a suggested energy maintenance routine that you can use to care for your energies on a daily basis.

Suggested Daily Energy Maintenance Routine

Morning:

1. On waking, become present in your body. Use the breathing and grounding exercises outlined earlier.
2. Visualize what goals you want to achieve today and how you want to feel by the end of the day.
3. Give gratitude in advance for this day.

4. Do a self-care check-in (see *Exercise 4-1: Self-Care Check-In* on page 83) to see what you need right now.

5. Cleanse your auric field using the Waterfall Cleanse or Aura Brushing exercise. You can do this while washing or taking a shower.

6. Charge your field using the Basic Charging exercise described earlier. Yoga or physical exercise is also good.

7. Eat a nutritious breakfast.

During the Day:

8. Do the check-in exercises at noon and anytime you feel knocked off balance.

9. Check how well you're achieving the goals that you visualized for the day in step 2.

10. If you're drifting from your goals, use grounding to become present, go into your bubble and make the necessary adjustments to your plans and choices.

11. Eat a nutritious lunch.

12. If possible, take a power nap after lunch or do some deep breathing and charging exercises (preferably outside) to refresh yourself for the afternoon.

13. Leave your work AT WORK and go home by 6 PM. See your work on your desk and physically or mentally close the door on it.

Evening:

14. After arriving home, clear your auric field using the Waterfall Cleanse or Aura Brushing technique to remove any negative energy that you may have picked up at work, on the bus or elsewhere.

15. After clearing, charge your field using the Basic Charging exercise described earlier. Yoga or physical exercise is also helpful.

16. Eat a nutritious (preferably home-cooked) dinner.

17. Relax and enjoy the company of family and friends.

Bedtime:

18. Go to bed before midnight (preferably before 11 PM). Choose a time that will allow you 7-8 hours of sleep before you have to get up. Make sure you allow time for your morning routine.

19. In bed, review the day with gratitude. List 10 things for which you're grateful.

20. As you become drowsy, breathe deeply and relax into the sensations of letting go and drifting into sleep.

Summary

The key to success when instilling new habits is practice. Start using the check-in exercises regularly until they become an automatic part of your day. Then practice the techniques you learned in this chapter to strengthen and maintain your energies.

As you try each technique out, keep using the check-in exercises to see how it affects you—experience is the best teacher. Eventually, energy maintenance will become an enjoyable and rewarding part of your day.

In the next chapter, you'll discover your natural energy cycles and you'll learn the art of successfully surfing your personal energy wave.

CHAPTER 6

Surfing Your Personal Energy Wave

When we breathe, inhaling is just as important as exhaling. And like our breathing, our energy has cycles of expansion and contraction, both of which are equally vital (see Figure 6-1).

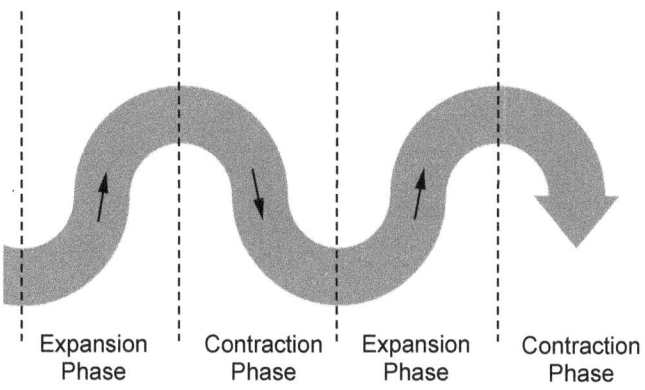

Figure 6-1: Personal Energy Wave Cycles

During the expansion phase, our energies build and move outward. This is a time of action, of movement and change, of connecting with others, of creative expression and of achievement. At the end of the expansion, our energies turn around and begin contracting inwards to recharge.

During the contraction phase, we integrate the effects of all that we experienced during the expansion. We sort out clutter, we analyze the past to learn lessons from our experiences, we reconnect to ourselves and we focus on healing and regeneration. The contraction energies prepare us to receive new creative ideas.

At the end of the contraction, our energy turns around and a new expansion phase begins. As the energy builds, we feel a natural desire to bring into the world those creative ideas that we received during the contraction phase. And so the cycle continues.

What Happens When We Fight Our Energy?

When we resist the direction that our energy is trying to take us, we create discomfort and stress in our lives. Our inner battle comes back to haunt us in our relationships, in our work, in our health and in our self-esteem.

Because of the active bias of our culture, we tend to resist contraction more than expansion. However, sometimes we may feel apprehensive and resist taking action, even though our energy is building in an expansion. This happens especially when we're facing a big change in our lives, like getting married.

This section describes some of the symptoms we can expect when we fight our cycle.

Resisting Expansion

If our energies are increasing, but we're resisting the expansion (perhaps because of fear of taking action), we may find ourselves:

- Discharging the extra energy through sexual activity, excessive talking or gossip, fighting, shopping, over-exercising, excessive partying, Internet surfing, or video games and so on
- Feeling bored or stuck
- Escaping into vicarious activity, such as watching sports on TV rather than playing a sport
- Procrastinating on tasks we know we should be doing
- Jumping from one topic or fad to another, rather than applying our energies toward a meaningful goal

If we're avoiding physical activity, we may find that our mental activity increases to compensate, leading to insomnia and lack of sleep. The next day, we feel too tired to move and the cycle worsens. Eventually, we may experience joint and muscle pain from inactivity.

Resisting Contraction

If we try to be active when our energies are in contraction, we may find ourselves:

- Having trouble staying motivated
- Subtly sabotaging ourselves at every turn
- Making careless mistakes
- Becoming clumsy and accident-prone
- Feeling irritable or depressed
- Wanting to sleep all the time
- Becoming more needy around others, wanting them to give us attention

We may also judge ourselves, which makes the contraction deepen. Self-judgment drains our energy, which means we have to go deeper to recharge it. If we do not stop the negative spiral, we may become ill. Colds, flu symptoms and digestive problems are common during a contraction phase; our bodies are forcing us to slow down.

Surfing Your Personal Energy Wave

When we fight our energy cycle, we set ourselves up for an energy crisis — we begin to feel burned out or drained. However, when we know how to work consciously with our personal energy wave, we can stay balanced no matter where in the cycle we find ourselves.

Here is how to surf your energy wave successfully.

Surfing the Peaks (Expansion Phase)

If your energy is in expansion:

- **Do vigorous physical activity**—You may be resisting the expansion in one aspect of your energy and not in others. For example, you may be resisting physical expansion, while allowing your energies to expand mentally or spiritually. Physical activity helps to spread the energy out into the other parts of your being.

- **Take the first step towards a dream or cherished goal**—This is especially helpful if you're procrastinating taking action because you feel overwhelmed. If you can take one small step in the right direction, the expanding energies will build and help motivate you to take the next step.

- **Use your energy wisely, while it's high**—Your energy is a precious resource. Now is the time to make productive use of it, rather than squandering it on tasks that are unimportant in the long run. Prioritize your tasks and tackle the most important ones first—those that really matter to you. You'll feel great for having completed them and you'll make forward progress toward the goals that add meaning to your life.

- **Connect with others**—Connect with people you appreciate and with whom you enjoy doing things together. It's also a great time for team building. When your energies are high you have a positive effect on others and will more easily inspire and motivate them to cooperate in your projects.

Surfing the Dips (Contraction Phase)

If your energy is in contraction:

- **Practice *being*, rather than *doing***—During a contraction, our energy moves naturally inwards causing a more introverted and reflective state of mind. Make use of this time for contemplation or reflection. You can also do a spiritual check-in to get insights on the big picture of your life.

    We access wisdom while simply being, rather than doing. This does not mean that we have to remain motionless. We can experience the state of being while we're moving, for example, when going for a walk in nature. It's just a matter of how we focus our conscious awareness. Mindfulness is the answer.

- **Clear the past**—Look for recurring patterns that create negative results in your life, for example always attracting partners who criticize you. These patterns point to an underlying subconscious belief at work. The contraction phase is a great time to work with a therapist, counselor or energy healer to release old patterns that no longer serve us. It's also a good time to get rid of old clutter that's keeping us from moving forward in our lives.

- **Increase your level of self-care**—The contraction phase is when we recharge our energies, so self-care is very important. Take the needed breaks from work or over-activity. If you have to go to work, make sure that you get enough sleep. Try to get to work earlier, rather than working later, if working late drains your energies.

Give yourself plenty of water and nourishing food. Eat slowly and enjoy your meals. Open your heart to your family, your friends and yourself. Do yoga and other slower, more relaxing, forms of exercise. You might want to schedule a detoxification cleanse, a fast or a retreat at this time. Massage is also good.

In other words, be kind to yourself. You'll find that going with the flow shortens the contraction phase and restores your energies much sooner and in a more pleasurable way. Then you're ready to move forward with the next expansion.

It's worth noting that the further we expand, the sooner our contraction will occur and the deeper it will go. Often people are dismayed when a day after making major progress in their work, a sport or a relationship, they suddenly find themselves feeling self-doubt or slipping up. What they don't realize is that their energy system is just shifting back to contraction mode. Because they are no longer charging ahead with their plans, they think that something is wrong with them and try to fix the situation.

The chief mistake here is slipping into self-judgment. Instead, it helps to shift into introspection and gentle curiosity. What might be going on here? Immediately ask yourself if you recently had an expansion experience. If so, then you're probably contracting and can relax knowing that is exactly what you're meant to do.

Take time off, if possible, for a day. If you have to go to work, focus on nondemanding tasks such as reports and basic chores that you put off when you were busy. We know this is not always easy to do in an office environment where deadlines are always looming. If possible, choose to work from home that day. You'll make fewer mistakes and will return to work sooner, with more energy and insights to spare.

The contraction phase is where our creativity gestates, if we let it. This is when we internally mull over problems that have been stopping us. Then creative solutions suddenly come to us, seemingly out of nowhere. That is the gift of the contraction phase.

So if you have some thorny problem that no amount of logic can make a dent in, put the problem aside until your next contraction—usually only a day or so away. Meanwhile, work on something else where you can make forward progress.

Where Are You in Your Energy Cycle?

It's helpful to know where we are in our energy cycle. In fact, this is a good thing to include as part of our regular energy check-in.

Each person is unique. If you keep an energy journal, you can see how your personal cycle works and get an idea of how long your contraction and expansion cycles typically last.

You can also keep track of what you did during the last expansion or contraction and learn from experience what activities work best in each part of your cycle.

Where are you in your energy cycle right now? Try the following exercise to find out.

Exercise 6-1: Mapping Your Personal Energy Wave

1. Put checkmarks in each column next to all the words that describe how you are feeling right now:

Expansion Signs	**Contraction Signs**
☐ Excited	☐ Peaceful
☐ Motivated	☐ Contemplative
☐ Analyzing	☐ Creating
☐ Active	☐ Resting
☐ Doing	☐ Being
☐ Communicative	☐ Quiet
☐ Mentally active	☐ Unfocussed or dreamy
☐ Logical	☐ Intuitive
☐ Extroverted	☐ Introverted
☐ Fast	☐ Slow
☐ Talking	☐ Listening
☐ Awake	☐ Sleepy
☐ Teaching	☐ Learning
☐ Giving	☐ Receiving
☐ Energized	☐ Tired
☐ Thinking about the future	☐ Reflecting on the past
____Total checked	____Total checked

2. Count the number of checkmarks in each column and write the total in the space provided. The column with the most checkmarks shows where you are in your energy cycle.

> 3. Ask yourself whether you're working with your energy cycle or resisting it.
> 4. What action, if any, do you need to take right now to bring yourself back in harmony with your personal energy wave?
> 5. What did you learn from this exercise? Make a note of your perceptions.
>
> **Note:** If your totals are equal or very similar, you may be in transition from one phase to the other. What is your intuitive sense about which direction your cycle is moving? Make a note of it. Then try the exercise again in a day or so to find out.

Summary

Managing your energy is like surfing a wave. It takes sensitivity and a fine sense of balance. In this chapter, you've learned how to work with your own energy cycle to stay balanced as your energy moves through its natural phases of expansion and contraction.

Practice checking in with your energy wave every day and making the proper adjustments to your self-care and activities to stay in harmony with your cycles.

Working with your own energy cycle is an important skill to master. But we don't live our lives in a vacuum. Subconscious patterns, relationships and daily events all have a powerful impact on us and can throw our energy out of balance. In the next chapter, you'll learn how to read the clues contained within your energy field to restore and balance your energies.

CHAPTER 7

Restoring Inner Balance

In our western culture, we rarely pay attention to the messages coming to us from our own energy senses about the imbalances in our bodies, in our relationships, in our environment and in how we live our lives. Unfortunately, if not dealt with, those imbalances eventually develop into health problems, relationship conflicts and other stressful events.

But if we learn how to pay attention to the energy messages we're receiving within, we can manage our energy in daily life situations so other people and external events are less likely to throw us off balance.

In Chapter 3, you learned how to become clear within so you could sense the state of your energy self. When you use the check-in exercises regularly, you can learn to identify energy imbalances in your life before they grow into larger problems.

An imbalance usually points to a situation where you're neglecting your own needs. In this chapter, you'll learn how to use the clues provided by your energy to decide what actions you need to take to return to balance quickly and easily.

Balancing Your Physical Energy

What can cause imbalances in our physical energy? Whenever we make changes to our physical habits, to our environment or when we experience hormonal changes, we'll experience upsets to our physical energy balance. Examples include:

- **Changes in diet**—A new diet or starting a detoxification program alters our metabolism and it may take some time to adapt.

- **Changes in sleep rhythms**—When we start working a night shift, suffer from jet lag or lose sleep because of a new baby, our biorhythms become confused and disoriented. We feel tired until our energy learns to adapt.

- **Injuries or illnesses**—Pain and discomfort, as well as the side effects of medications, can interfere with the flow of our energy. Our routines are also disrupted by reduced mobility or hospitalization.

- **Weather or seasonal changes**—Rainy or hot, humid weather conditions tend to drain our energy. In some countries, long dark winters can cause seasonal affective disorder (SAD) and vitamin D deficiency.

- **Hormonal changes**—Our hormonal balance can shift because of PMS, puberty, childbirth, menopause, andropause (the male version of menopause) or thyroid problems, upsetting our physical energy.

In addition, any major stresses in the emotional, mental and spiritual areas of our being will also affect our physical energies.

Physical Balancing Messages

Physical sensations are the instrument panel of our body. Just as we would be foolish to ignore the engine oil warning light in our car, it's equally foolish to ignore our physical discomfort. If we ignore it or try to numb it with medication, the underlying problem doesn't go away—it gets worse.

Only we know what life imbalance is causing our own particular physical problem. And that information is available to us when we're willing to check into our own energy field. Our physical energy gives us messages in the form of symptoms when the balance is off. These symptoms provide clues about what we need to do to return to balance. The table in *Appendix A: Physical Balancing Messages* shows some of the most common physical balancing messages and provides suggestions for returning to balance.

Restoring Your Physical Energy Balance

When your physical energy balance is off, how can you get back into balance? First, notice the imbalance. Typically, you'll feel some physical symptom.

Next, find out what this symptom is trying to tell you. You can sense it intuitively or look up your symptom in *Appendix A: Physical Balancing Messages* and see if the suggested message feels true for you.

Finally, take action to correct the underlying cause suggested by the message. You may need to make changes in your life situation or in how you perceive it. If the problem is lack of self-care, take immediate steps to look after your own needs.

If a physical symptom is pointing to an issue on the emotional, mental or spiritual level, a simple attitude change may be all you need to change the situation into an opportunity for healing.

For more stubborn issues, you might need the help of a therapist to work through it. For example, if you find yourself getting sick a lot, you may find that you have a subconscious belief that being sick gets you sympathy and love. If being ill is the only way for you to get love in your life, you may find it hard to change the pattern. A therapist or energy practitioner can help you to resolve it.

The following exercise will give you some practice in sensing your physical balancing messages and discovering what steps you need to take to return to balance physically.

Exercise 7-1: Restoring Your Physical Energy Balance

Have paper and pen handy to record notes.

1. Find a comfortable position and close your eyes.
2. Bring your attention to your breathing.
3. Take in a deep breath and let it out with a sigh. Repeat this three times.
4. Take another deep breath and allow your awareness to sink into the body.
5. Ask yourself the following questions:
   - Which part of my body is calling for my attention right now?
   - What sensations am I feeling in that part of my body?
   - What message does that part of my body want to tell me?
   - What does that part of my body need right now to feel better?
   - What changes do I need to make in my self-care to return to physical balance in this part of my body?
6. When finished, take another deep breath and let it out with a sigh.
7. Open your eyes and make a note of what you learned.

Balancing Your Emotional Energy

Many things can upset our emotional balance, including:

- **Low physical energy**—When our physical vitality is drained due to poor health, hunger or fatigue, for example, we become more emotionally dependent on others. Our dependency creates a power imbalance in our relationship with them, which makes us more vulnerable to emotional upset.

- **Emotional stress or shock**—Emotional stress and shock also affect our emotional balance. For example, if we've received the shocking news of the death or injury of a loved one, it will upset us greatly and take precedence over our other normal emotions. Also, long-term emotional stress, for example, dealing with an abusive or alcoholic spouse, can overload our emotional energies to the point of burnout. This affects all the other levels of our energy, as well.

- **Arguments and interactions with others**—For most of us, arguments and interactions with others are a frequent source of emotional energy upsets. Our loved ones may "push our buttons" when they behave in ways that evoke painful experiences from our own childhood. For example, Fred's parents ignored his opinions when he was a child, which made him feel unimportant and invisible. Now when his spouse makes decisions without consulting him, he gets very upset.

- **Repressed emotions**—We tend to be unaware of repressed emotional energy, because it stays hidden until we're triggered by something that reminds us of the original trauma. Then the emotion suddenly comes to the surface, seemingly out of nowhere. A clue that we may be dealing with repressed emotional energy is when our reaction is out of proportion to the situation.

- **Mental judgments**—Our mental judgments can also upset our emotional energy balance. In fact, it's what we tell ourselves that typically causes our emotional reactions to the people and events around us.

    Many of our thoughts are so habitual that they happen too quickly for us to notice and we react as if by instinct. But if we look closely, we'll discover that we did tell ourselves something. Often our minds may have interpreted an event or situation as a personal threat. For example, we see a person we know standing across the street at a busy intersection. Just as we wave at them, they turn and walk away. We feel rejected. The thoughts go something like this: "Hey! They deliberately ignored me! What did I do wrong?" In truth, the person may have just turned away because they suddenly remembered an errand in the other direction. These sorts of misunderstandings happen all the time, simply because of the chatter in our heads.

- **Someone else's energy**—Sometimes we can feel an emotion for no obvious reason. For example, we may be happy one moment. Then the phone rings and after we hang up, we feel depressed. What may have happened is that we picked up someone else's energy. We don't even have to be in contact with them. Just thinking of them can bring on an emotion.

   When the emotions we feel are not ours, it means that we've picked up some unwanted energy and that it's time to clear the energy field using one of the techniques on pages 121–126 in Chapter 5, *Maintaining Your Energy*.

Emotional Balancing Messages

Emotions tell us about the power balance in our lives. We need to pay attention to them. Our painful emotions are messages that tell us when our emotional balance is off.

   The table in *Appendix B: Emotional Balancing Messages* describes the most common emotional balancing messages and provides suggestions for returning to balance.

Restoring Your Emotional Energy Balance

It's just as unhealthy to let our emotions run riot as it is to repress them. So, what is a healthy way to express our emotions? If we know how to handle emotional energy, we simply allow ourselves to feel it and explore it.

The art of exploring our emotional messages involves the delicate balance of fully experiencing our emotions, including their physical impact such as heart rate, sweating or clamminess, while staying calmly detached as the observer and paying attention to what else is going on. What was the thought just preceding our feeling? What would we have to believe to think that way?

The healing of the underlying pattern happens naturally as a result of the conscious exploration. The key is not to make the emotion go away, but rather to listen to its message with kind curiosity. It wants to speak to us. That is its purpose—to get our attention and direct us to a perceived problem. It is a marvelous self-healing mechanism.

It helps to remember that our emotions are energy. We can think of each emotion as a frequency of energy, like a particular color is a frequency of light.

The following exercise will give you some practice in interpreting your emotional balancing messages and discovering what steps you need to take to return to balance.

Note: If more than one emotion is coming up at a time, we suggest taking the time to work through each one individually, rather than trying to work through all of them at the same time. With practice, this process will become easier and you'll be able to resolve your emotional balance quickly. You can also use this process when working with a therapist.

Exercise 7-2: Restoring Your Emotional Energy Balance

Have paper and pen handy to record notes.

1. Sit in a comfortable position and close your eyes.
2. Bring your attention to your breathing.
3. Take in a deep breath and let it out with a sigh. Repeat this three times.
4. Allow your awareness to go inward and tune into your emotions. Is any emotion calling for your attention right now? If so, allow your awareness to be with that emotion.
5. If the emotion is a sudden shift from what you were feeling before, ask yourself the following questions:

    - What was I doing just before the shift? For example, was I reading, watching TV, chatting with someone or riding the bus?
    - What was I thinking about?
    - What was I telling myself?
    - Is this my energy or could I be picking up someone else's energy?

6. If the energy feels like it belongs to someone else, then use the Aura Brushing technique to clear your field of their energies. (See *Exercise 5-10: Aura Brushing* on page 122.)

7. If the energy is your own and you're someplace where you can safely express the emotion, then do the following:

    - Allow yourself to simply notice and experience the emotion.

    - If the emotion produces discomfort, do not resist or fight it, just stay with the energy.

    - Express the emotion as necessary—cry, scream or hit a pillow, for example.

    - The energy will change. Stay with the experience and watch where it takes you. Notice the shifts in perspective and insights that come to you after the emotional release.

8. Allow the energy to resolve itself. The balancing message will reveal itself if you're patient and willing to learn from the situation.

9. Open your eyes and make a note of what you learned.

10. If the emotional release was particularly powerful, you will probably need to contract afterwards. Be kind to yourself— go for a walk in nature, or have a nice long relaxing bath, for example. (See Chapter 6, *Surfing Your Personal Energy Wave* for more information on how to support yourself during an energy contraction.)

Note: If you're unable to resolve the emotion on your own, then consult a therapist who can help you with this. You can also look up the emotion in *Appendix B: Emotional Balancing Messages* and, if it feels right for you, try the suggested advice.

Balancing Your Mental Energy

Our energies interact. Many of the things described earlier that upset our physical or emotional balance, usually also affect our mental balance. Other things that can upset our mental balance include:

- **Mind-altering substances**—drugs, medications and alcohol
- **Mental illness**—chronic depression, bipolar disorder, schizophrenia and others
- **Mental shock and trauma**—mental isolation or abuse, brainwashing, post-traumatic stress syndrome
- **Work stress**—deadlines, excessive responsibilities or overwork
- **Spiritual issues**—loss of faith, lack of direction or meaning, lack of conscience

Mental Balancing Messages

When our mental energy is out of balance, the first thing we may lose is our sense of humor. We become very serious and tend to take things personally. We may feel confused and stressed by life and other people.

Some of us may find ourselves becoming perfectionists and driven to obsess over details. Others of us may escape into fantasies or addictions to avoid dealing with our problems. If taken to the extreme, any of these reactions may cause our lives to fall apart around us, resulting in divorce, debt or physical problems, for example.

As we can see, allowing our mental energy to go too far out of balance can have dramatic, stressful and sometimes tragic results in our lives. However, we can learn to read the inner balancing messages that our mental energy is giving us well in advance and then take suitable steps to restore our mental energy balance before it affects our lives so dramatically. *Appendix C: Mental Balancing Messages* describes some of the most common balancing messages at the mental energy level and provides suggestions on what actions to take to come into balance.

Restoring Your Mental Energy Balance

Everything we need to come back into balance is available to us within our own energy, when we learn how to notice and interpret our mental balancing messages. Deep inside, we know what we need for health and sanity.

The following exercise will give you some practice in interpreting your mental balancing messages and discovering what steps you need to take to restore your mental energy balance.

Note: If more than one mental pattern is coming up at a time, we suggest taking the time to work through each one individually, rather than trying to work through all of them at the same time. With practice, this process will become easier and you'll be able to resolve your mental balance quickly. You can also use this process when working with a therapist.

Exercise 7-3: Restoring Your Mental Energy Balance

Have paper and pen handy to record notes.

1. Sit in a comfortable position and close your eyes.
2. Bring your attention to your breathing.
3. Take in a deep breath and let it out with a sigh. Repeat this three times.
4. Allow your awareness to go inward and tune into your thoughts.
5. Ask yourself the following questions:

   - What discomfort (if any) are my thoughts giving me right now?
   - What situation in my life is causing those thoughts?
   - What message is my discomfort trying to tell me about this situation?
   - How does the situation need to change in order for me to feel better about it?
   - What attitude would I need to have to create the situation I want? Am I willing to try changing my attitude right now?
   - From this new attitude, what ideas occur to me for resolving this problem? What actions do I need to take in alignment with this new attitude?

- What small step am I willing to take in the direction I want?
- Can I take that small step today?

6. When finished, take another deep breath and let it out with a sigh.
7. Open your eyes and make a note of what you learned.

Note: If you're unable to resolve your mental state on your own, you may need to consult a therapist who can help you with this. You can also look up the mental pattern in *Appendix C: Mental Balancing Messages* and, if it feels right for you, try the suggested advice.

Balancing Your Spiritual Energy

What causes us to lose our spiritual balance? Experiences that affect our physical, emotional and mental energy balance, often affect our spiritual balance as well. Other things that can upset our spiritual energy balance include:

- Ignoring conscience or intuition
- Excessive worrying and focusing on problems to the exclusion of all else
- Excessive focus on material things
- Refusing to give or receive love
- Blocked creativity or self-expression
- Dishonesty or deceitful behavior

- Lost contact with self (because we have no time or we're too busy, for example)
- Excessive self-absorption to the exclusion of other people

Spiritual Balancing Messages

Our spiritual energy is our inner guidance system for leading a fulfilled and meaningful life. When we ignore our spiritual balancing messages, they get louder. Eventually, they cause a crisis in our lives that we can no longer ignore. Examples include such things as illness, accidents, relationship troubles, betrayal, deception and nervous breakdown.

After a crisis occurs, it's much harder to return to balance—our energy systems are overwhelmed and our health may be compromised. When our energy is low, it's difficult to stay positive and to see clearly to find solutions to our problems.

However, if we notice the imbalance while it's still minor, then we can use our energy skills to return to balance quickly and avert a crisis. The table in *Appendix D: Spiritual Balancing Messages* describes some of the most common balancing messages at the spiritual energy level and suggested steps for restoring balance.

Restoring Your Spiritual Energy Balance

Once you've decided that your spiritual energy is out of balance, how can you restore it quickly? The exercise that follows will give you an experience of how to restore your spiritual energy balance.

Note: If more than one pattern is coming up at a time, we suggest taking the time to work through each one individually, rather than trying to work through all of them at the same time. With practice, this process will become easier and you'll be able to restore your spiritual balance quickly. You can also use this process when working with a therapist or spiritual counselor.

Exercise 7-4: Restoring Your Spiritual Energy Balance

Have paper and pen handy to record notes.

1. Find a comfortable position and close your eyes.
2. Bring your attention to your breathing.
3. Take in a deep breath and let it out with a sigh. Repeat this 3 times.
4. Allow your awareness to go inward and tune into your spiritual energy.
5. Ask yourself the following questions:

    - What discomfort (if any) am I experiencing right now in my spirit?

    - What situation might be causing that discomfort?

    - What is my intuitive sense or gut feeling telling me about the situation?

    - What is my part in the situation? How am I making it worse?

    - What could I do instead to turn this into a win-win scenario for

> all concerned?
> - Am I willing to do my part?
> - What do I truly want to experience in this moment? What is my heart telling me right now? What are my dreams telling me right now?
> - What small step can I take now in this direction?
>
> 6. When finished, take another deep breath and let it out with a sigh.
> 7. Open your eyes and make a note of what you learned.
>
> **Note:** If you're unable to resolve the spiritual issue on your own, you may need to consult a therapist or spiritual counselor who can help you with this. You can also look up the symptom in *Appendix D: Spiritual Balancing Messages* and, if it feels right for you, try the suggested advice.

Summary

As with any skill, practice makes perfect. Make it a new habit to notice how you're feeling at any given time in the physical, emotional, mental or spiritual parts of your energy self. When you become aware of discomfort in any of these areas, use the skills you've just learned to bring yourself into balance.

You might consider keeping a journal of what comes up, how you dealt with it and what was the result. That way, you'll begin to learn how to interpret what your own balancing messages mean. When you're feeling badly, don't beat yourself up about it. Just notice that you're out of balance and at that moment apply the techniques.

Eventually, they will become second nature to you. In the next chapter, we'll explore how to use energy awareness to create a fulfilling and balanced life.

Part III

Taking Your Energy into the World

CHAPTER 8

Energy and Your Life

Our life balance reflects the degree to which we feel fulfilled in our lives. When our lives are balanced in all areas, it means that we're expressing ourselves fully in each area, no one area is dominating our experience or being neglected.

Like our energy bodies, when we block our energy from full expression in any area of our lives, we experience growing stress and frustration. If not addressed, the problems in the neglected area worsen until they lead to a crisis, which can eventually affect other areas such as our health and relationships.

When we identify where we're not fully expressing ourselves in our lives, we can learn to use our energies in new ways to bring those areas back into balance so our lives work for us, rather than against us. This chapter provides the tools to do this.

How Do Our Lives Get Out of Balance?

Our life balance, like our energy, is not static. We may feel more balanced at some times in our lives than at other times. Any major life event that forces us to change our habits, can throw us off balance:

- **Changes in marital status**—Getting married or becoming newly single

- **Added responsibilities**—Becoming a parent or caring for an invalid

- **Changes in employment**—Starting a new job, being promoted, losing your job, starting a business or retiring

- **Increased financial burdens**—Buying a home or starting college

- **Moving homes**—Adapting to a different city or country

- **Changes in physical health**—Becoming ill or disabled

- **External events**—War, political upheaval, economic recession or natural disasters

Apart from major life changes and external events, our own habitual reactions to stress can also lead to an unbalanced life. Examples of habitual reactions that can lead to life imbalances include:

- **Denial**—We ignore the problems in our lives. We pretend that they don't exist or hope that they will go away by themselves. Unaddressed, the problems get worse and eventually build into a major crisis, for example, we ignore physical pain symptoms until we need an operation.

- **Procrastination**—We recognize that our problems exist, but we put off dealing with them until a crisis erupts.

- **Lack of clarity**—Unrealistic about our abilities or future goals, we fail to plan properly and we make faulty decisions that result in disappointments or losses in one or more areas of our lives.

- **Lack of connection to self**—When we lose contact with the self, perhaps through over-giving in relationship, we lose our awareness of our real needs, neglecting them. Over time, this creates inner stress, which eventually erupts in a crisis.

- **Irresponsibility or excessive responsibility**—When we refuse to take responsibility for our own actions, it keeps us in a childish mind-set. We blame others for all that is wrong in our lives, not realizing that our own behavior is causing our problems. Conversely, when we assume excessive responsibility for others, for example over-parenting grown-up children, we not only deprive our children of valuable life experiences, but we also deprive ourselves of the time we need for our own fulfillment.

- **Self-indulgence and addictions**—Self-indulgence is a substitute for true self-care. It eventually results in a depletion of energy or money. Self-indulgence can easily become an addiction when it serves as an escape from our lives. Escapism has the same result as denial—the problems in our lives multiply until a crisis occurs.

- **Inflexibility**—Our life circumstances constantly change. That is the very nature of life. If we're unable to adapt to change, we react with old behaviors that do not work and our lives become stressed and unbalanced as a result.

How Do We Know When Our Lives Are Out Of Balance?

Sometimes we're so busy living our lives that we're unaware that they are out of balance. Usually it takes a strong message, shock or crisis to get our attention and to force us to take action. Here are some common clues that can point to life balance problems:

- Chronic pain, fatigue or illness
- Feeling overwhelmed or procrastinating
- Addictions or escapism
- Personal crises or drama
- Loss of sense of humor

- Workaholism
- Irritability
- Co-dependency
- Disorganized or chaotic home environment

How Can We Restore Balance in Our Lives?

Balancing our lives is not about treating ourselves as a commodity to be distributed—20% here, 40% there, for example. It's about becoming a whole person. It is about treating ourselves lovingly in all areas of our lives to achieve wholeness.

Just as it's important to be fully present in our bodies and our energy fields for health and well-being, it's equally important to be fully present in every area of our lives. Those places in our lives where we feel lack or dissatisfaction are the very places where we're not fully present with ourselves and with what is happening in the moment.

To restore balance in our lives, we start by becoming aware of what is happening in each area. Wherever we feel unfulfilled, we must look at how our behaviors and actions are contributing to the situation. We identify what needs and expectations are important to us in that area and that we're not meeting. Finally, we explore what changes we need to make to feel fulfilled in that life area.

Figure 8-1 shows the twelve life areas that most of us feel are important to our happiness and fulfillment.

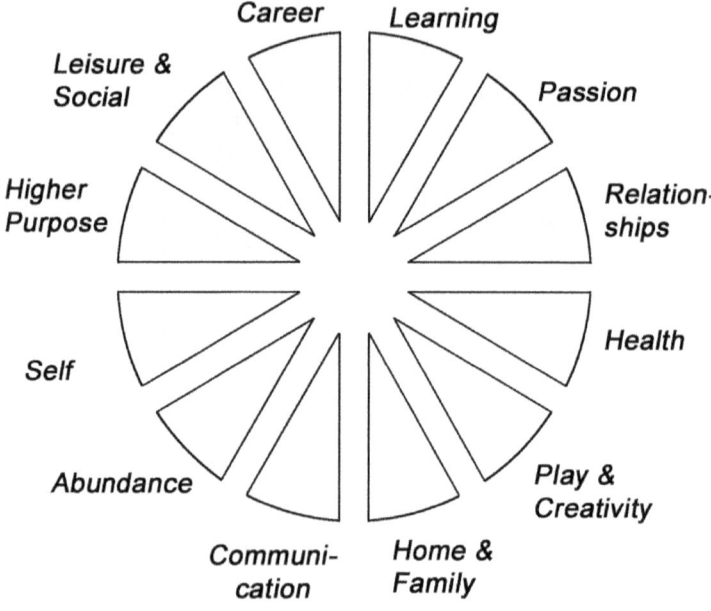

Figure 8-1: Life Balance Areas

Let's take a look at what we need for balance and fulfillment in each area:

Self

This life area encompasses our relationship with the self, including our awareness of our feelings, thoughts, beliefs, our self-esteem, our personal power, our dreams and goals, our gifts and abilities and our conscience. It also represents the degree to which we take responsibility for our own well-being.

When we're not fully present in the area of the Self, we depend on others and external things for our sense of self-worth. We create situations where we get confused or hurt, or take things personally, because we rely on others to make us feel good about ourselves. Then we blame them for what is wrong in our lives.

However, when we're present and aware in this area, we're able to stay connected with ourselves even when we're with other people. We pay attention to the inner messages coming from our physical, emotional, mental and spiritual energies and we respond as needed with the proper self-care. We pay attention to our dreams, longings and conscience. And we trust in the wisdom of our hearts to guide us towards creating fulfillment in our lives.

Abundance

This life area reflects our ability to create the quality of life and attract the things and situations that we want, as well as our ability to appreciate what we do have. Abundance is closely tied in with our personal energy levels and our sense of self-worth. Abundance is more than just the amount of money we have. It also represents an expansive sense of freedom and well-being— a sense of unlimited possibilities and of having many choices available to us in our lives.

When we're not fully present in this area, we usually feel deprived in some way. We focus on what is missing rather than feeling grateful for how abundance appears in other ways in our lives. For example, if we have plenty of money, we fear losing it. Or perhaps we decide we need more. If we have no money, we allow that to be a reason not to enjoy what we do have, such as good health or loving relationships.

However, when we're fully present in the area of Abundance, we're grateful for what we have, and care for our belongings with respect and appreciation. We take responsibility for our financial health and are willing to look at our current situation closely and clearly. We notice how our standard of living affects our energy and take suitable action to make those changes necessary for our well-being.

Communication

This life area reflects our ability to express ourselves and understand others. It also represents our ability to ask for what we need and to negotiate.

When we're not fully present in this area, we often experience confusion and misunderstandings in our dealings with others. Others don't listen to us. They don't give us what we want because we don't know how to ask for it. People get upset with us for no obvious reason. We may feel alone and unable to bridge the gap to connect with others. Others may not trust us, or vice versa. We may not communicate honestly, perhaps putting on a happy face to hide our pain.

However, when we're fully present in the area of Communication, we're able to look at our communications objectively and to see our own role in creating any misunderstandings that occur. We're willing to learn new ways of communicating to reduce misunderstandings. We become able to listen to others and ourselves effectively.

Home and Family

This life area reflects how we feel about our home environment, our personal sanctuary or safe haven within which we protect, support and nurture ourselves and our loved ones. It also represents our relationships with those who live with us, including our children, parents, spouses, partners or roommates who with us create the emotional energy of our home environment.

When we're not fully present in this area of our lives, we tend to stay away from our home as much as possible. Our withdrawal may be the result of a toxic emotional environment in the home. If we live by ourselves, it may be our fear of being alone with our own thoughts that keeps us away. Either way, avoiding the issue only makes it worse. We may become workaholics. We may become strangers to our family members.

Our home may suffer from neglect, as we procrastinate doing our maintenance and chores. The chaos and mess in our surroundings further adds to our stress. Our feelings of being overwhelmed then spill out into other areas of our lives. If we're unable to relax at home, our moods and our health may eventually decline.

However, when we engage fully in area of Home and Family, we make the necessary effort to create a safe and welcoming home environment. We consider such things as the physical requirements of our home, cleanliness, warmth, comfort, space, the right mix of freedom and closeness and the sharing of chores.

We know that a harmonious emotional environment provides each member of the household with a lasting sense of safety and support, which strengthens them for dealing with the outside world. So we make the time to appreciate and to build relationships with each person who shares our home with us. We also stay true to ourselves and express our own needs, while connecting from the heart with others in our home.

Play and Creativity

This life sector reflects our ability to let go of our preconceived ideas and to open to new ideas, experiences, inspirations and forms of creative expression that expand our very sense of who we are. We can play with our children, our pets, other adults or we can play by ourselves.

During play, we relax, move our bodies more freely, laugh and express ourselves easily. Our serious adult masks drop away and we feel light and happy. In this playful state, we sense beauty and joy around us, as well as within us.

We have full access to our imaginations and creative inspiration flows easily. We can't help but want to share our unique expression of self with the world, whether in words, music, poetry, dance, art or some other form of creative expression that moves us. And in turn, creatively expressing this deepest, most essential part of ourselves fills us with energy and joy.

When we're not fully present in this life area, we tend to dismiss play as silly and childish. We may believe that we're just not creative. We become serious and critical of the creative attempts of others. We lose our sense of fun and enjoyment in life. We feel jaded. Life becomes hard work.

However, when we're fully present in the area of Play and Creativity, we make time for play and for our own unique creative expression, even if it means getting up earlier in the day. We listen to creative impulses arising from within and follow through on them. We honor our creativity by getting the training or guidance needed to help it flower into fullest expression. We lovingly protect our creations from premature criticism and analysis (including our own) until we're ready to share them with the world.

Health

This life area reflects our state of physical, emotional, mental and spiritual health and our ability to care for ourselves. It also reflects how aware we are of our needs and of what it takes to maintain our energies.

When we're not fully present in this life area, we tend to neglect our self-care and as a result suffer from energy depletion. Lower energy eventually leads to health problems and affects our abilities to make good decisions in other areas of our lives. We tend to ignore the inner balancing messages coming to us from our bodies, emotions, thoughts and conscience. Unaddressed, the underlying conditions continue to build into the future crises and upsets in our lives.

When we're fully present in the life area of Health, we take responsibility for properly feeding, exercising and caring for our physical bodies and energy fields. We consistently maintain our self-care for maximum health. We notice our inner balancing messages and respond suitably as needed. We live in harmony with our energy cycles, benefiting from contraction as well as expansion experiences. When necessary, we seek professional help to address any health problems.

Relationships

This life area reflects our ability to interact enjoyably with other people. It includes our ability to appreciate the unique contributions that other people bring to our lives, including love, other perspectives, ideas, fun, intimacy and companionship.

When we're not fully present in this life area, our relationships are few and unsatisfactory. We may become so self-absorbed with our own troubles that we do not recognize the help and support that may be available to us from others. We fail to see the role we play in sabotaging our relationships. We may love conditionally, withholding our love unless others do what we ask or love us in certain ways. Or else we may try to give too much in our relationships, hoping to earn love from others. However, our hidden demand for love taints our giving and we find people backing away from us instead. We may lose contact with our own loving nature, and begin to feel cold and bitter inside, blaming it on the failure of others to love us properly.

However, when we're fully present in the life area of Relationships, we appreciate and love other people. We learn how to accept others for who they are, rather than for whom we want them to be. We seek to create win-win situations in our relationships, where all parties benefit. We learn how to give and receive love. We treat others and ourselves with respect. We make the effort to get to know our children and our partners, and to be aware of what is going on in their lives, including their challenges and problems. We pay attention to what conclusions our children are drawing about life and we offer encouragement and loving guidance to them where needed.

Passion

This life sector represents how much passion, romance, stimulation, adventure and excitement we have in our lives. Passion is the "juice" of life. If we don't have something that excites us and keeps us enthusiastically involved, then life becomes boring and we wonder, "What's the point?" Whatever stimulates our passion has an element of the unknown or an element of risk that spices up our lives. Doing what we love opens our minds to new creative possibilities. Our passion inevitably takes us on a journey towards deeper purpose and meaning in our lives.

When we're not fully present in this area, our lives may feel boring and uninspired. We may seek fulfillment in external accomplishments or material things, but find ourselves disappointed when we achieve them. Then we chase after new goals, possessions or partners, hoping that they will provide the missing ingredient. When we're out of touch with our passion, or are avoiding it because of childhood conditioning, we may feel numbed and depressed. We may become addicted to substances or experiences that give us a temporary sense of aliveness, but cause our lives to spiral out of balance.

However, when we're fully present in the life area of Passion, we recognize that our deepest and most fulfilling passion comes from within as we get to know and express our true self into the world. We take responsibility for exploring what our deepest longing is and for responding to the opportunities that life sends us for fulfilling that longing.

Learning

This life area represents our ability to learn and apply information. It includes not only formal education, but also how well we learn from our life experiences and from our mistakes. Learning opens us to fresh opportunities. We learn skills, grow in awareness and understanding and meet new people. Each one of these experiences can change the direction of our lives.

When we're not fully present in this area, we find ourselves repeating the same old mistakes, because we keep making the same decisions in each situation. Unable to grow from our experiences or to develop new skills, we find ourselves becoming stale—old before our time, as our habits crystallize into rigid rules for living. We become blind to opportunities to improve our lives, because we can only see things one way. Then we are easily knocked off balance by the inevitable changes that life sends us.

When we're fully present in the Learning sector, we constantly seek to improve our skills and knowledge. We see every situation as an opportunity to learn more about others and ourselves. We realize there is no such thing as failure, only results. And we learn from the results of our choices, and keep adapting our approach each time the situation arises until we succeed. We realize that life keeps giving us new opportunities to discover and express who we really are and to lead fulfilling lives.

Career

This life area reflects not only what we do to earn a living, but also how we personally grow and develop through the work that we do. This can include the new skills and abilities that we learn as we gain experience from various jobs, such as technical skills or the ability to manage and motivate people. It can also include developing our sense of confidence in what we bring into the world. Our work can be a training ground for preparing us to move into our passion later.

When we're not fully present in this life sector, we find our work to be draining and unfulfilling. We may see our work as just a means to earn enough money to do other things. We may just do the minimum to keep our job or we may use our work to hide out from relationship problems. We may skip from job to job trying to find satisfaction or more money, but the same problems occur wherever we go.

However, when we're fully present in the Career area, we know that work occupies much of our time and so we want our work life to be satisfying and interesting. We choose a career or work that will provide opportunities for expressing our talents and abilities into the world. We explore what we're good at or what we long to be good at. We get the training we need to be able to do what we love full-time. We commit to strengthening our abilities and skills to take our work to its highest expression.

Leisure and Social Life

This life area reflects how we find relaxation, fun, enjoyment and mental stimulation—alone, as well as with others. Our social lives provide opportunities for such things as developing friendships, appreciating culture, enjoying food and sharing activities with others. We all need something that keeps us from being too self-absorbed. Our social and leisure pursuits bring us into the wider world, where we connect with new ideas and experiences.

When we're not fully present in this life area, we may find ourselves going along with others without really considering whether our social lives support who we are or what we need. For example, if we're trying to cut out smoking and drinking and our friends are all smokers and drinkers, we may find it a lot harder to give up these habits. Some of us may choose not to have a social life at all and instead stay home and watch TV much of the time. We may be so tense that we're unable to relax and enjoy ourselves alone or with other people.

However, when we're fully present in this life sector, we're aware of whether our social lives support who we really are and what we want in our lives. We choose activities and groups that are in harmony with what is important to us. We make time to take part in activities that we enjoy, make new friends and balance our socializing with quality time for ourselves.

Purpose

This life area reflects our sense of the larger purpose and meaning of our lives, including a sense of direction and a sense of contributing in some way to the larger world.

When we're not fully present in this area, we may feel that our lives are in a muddle or that we're going in circles. We may not have a clear idea of what we want to do, and our life experience may feel shallow and meaningless.

When we're fully present in the life area of Purpose, our lives are in alignment and integrity with who we really are. We feel we're heading in the right direction. When we're living "on purpose", we find our energies becoming strong and clear. We seek to direct our talents and abilities where they can most benefit others and ourselves. We find that our energy and way of being automatically begins to attract others who want to support us in our goals. The plight of humanity touches our hearts and we look for ways of making the world a better place.

How Balanced is Your Life?

The degree of balance in our lives reflects the degree to which we've grown up into healthy functioning adults, able to meet our responsibilities, while creating a meaningful and rewarding life.

Charting Your Life Balance

Here is an exercise to evaluate where you feel most fulfilled in your life and what areas still need further development for you to achieve balance.

Exercise 8-1: Your Life Balance Chart

For this exercise, you'll need two colored pens or pencils (one lighter and one darker.)

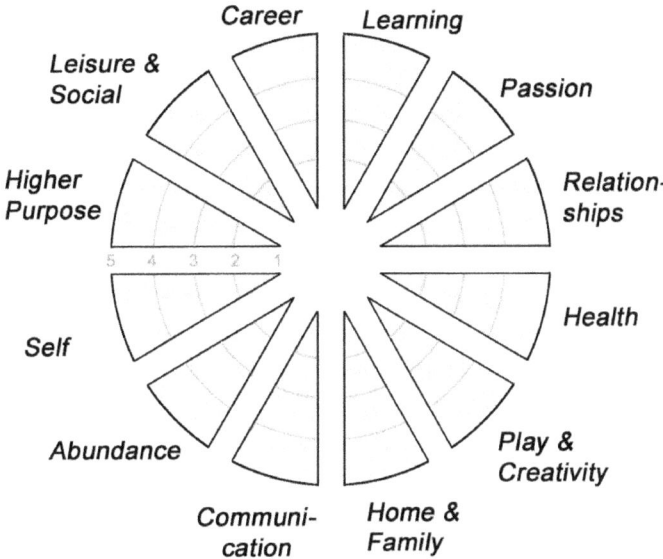

1. Using the lighter color and starting from the center, fill in each life area to the circle that marks how fulfilled you feel in that area of your life as follows:

   5 = Excellent (full), 4 = Very good, 3 = Good, 2 = Fair and
   1 = Poor (empty)

2. Using the darker color, place a dot in each slice of the life pie on the circle that marks how much time and energy you spend in that area of your life as follows:

   5 = Very large amount, 4 = More than average, 3 = Average,
   2 = Less than average, 1 = Little or none.

Analyzing Your Life Balance Chart

Before evaluating your life balance, it helps to balance your inner energy first, using the techniques in Chapter 7, *Restoring Inner Balance*. This will enable you to look at the outer events of your life objectively, rather than judging yourself or trying to blame others.

Any place that feels unfulfilled in your life will affect your energy. Like the different aspects of your personal energy field, the different life areas interact and sometimes compete. *Figure 8-2* shows an example of a completed life chart.

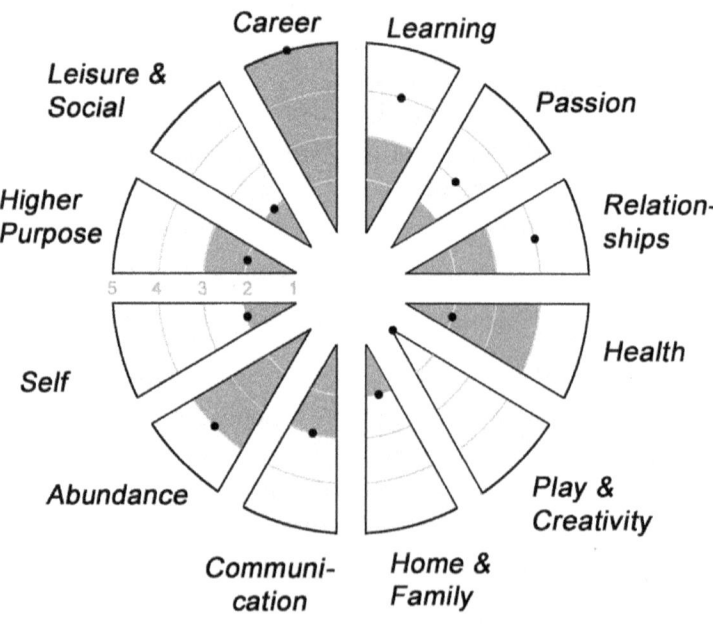

Figure 8-2: Example of Completed Life Chart

It's helpful to analyze your life chart with the following questions in mind:

- Looking at the overall chart, how balanced does it look in terms of fulfillment? Which areas are mostly empty or less than half-full (rating less than 3)? These areas represent opportunities for more fulfillment and happiness in your life. They are places where you need to restore wholeness in your life.

- In which area do you feel most fulfilled? Are there some skills or abilities that you can use from this area of your life that can help you in a less fulfilling area? Is there a way of combining the two areas through a common activity?

    For example, you may feel unfulfilled in the area of Family, maybe not spending as much time with your children as you would like. Perhaps you could involve your children in the health, creativity or leisure areas of your life to help improve your relationships with them.

- Looking at the overall chart, how balanced does it look in terms of where you spend your time and energy? Are you distributing your energy evenly in the various areas of your life, or are you spending too much energy in some areas and too little in others? Sometimes we focus our energies on what is easier in our lives as a way of avoiding what is more difficult for us. For example, the chart in *Figure 8-2* suggests someone whose excessive focus on their career may be an attempt to avoid facing problems at home.

- If there is an obvious imbalance in how you spend your time and energy:

  - Where are you spending the least time and energy (dots closest to the center)? Is there any issue that you might be avoiding in that area of your life (for example, lack of confidence, lack of ability or lack of time for yourself)?

  - Where are you spending the most time and energy (dots closer to the edge)? Are you possibly using those areas as an escape from another more troublesome area of your life?

- Is there any correlation between where you spend your time and energy and the amount of fulfillment that you feel in that area?

  - If the dot is located inside the shaded area of the slice, you're getting back more fulfillment than the energy you're spending. This life area is a net source of energy. For example, the chart in *Figure 8-2* shows that the person's excellent health and sense of purpose fuels their life with energy.

  - If the dot is located outside the shaded area, you're spending more time and energy than you're getting back in fulfillment. This area is a net energy drain. For example, the chart in *Figure 8-2* suggests that the person gives too much in the area of relationships and as a result may feel burdened or unsupported by others.

- If you're already spending a lot of time and energy in an area where you feel unfulfilled or frustrated, ask yourself whether you need to use a different approach or take another look at your goals. You could be trying to achieve a goal that is in conflict with what you really need and want.

For example, you may spend a lot of time trying to improve family relations, but it's not working and this is draining you. Maybe you need to let go and stop trying to control the situation. Pouring in more time and energy in the same old ways may not be the answer. Getting professional help through a family therapist or seeking some other form of support might be more effective.

Restoring Balance in Your Life

As you look at your own life balance, ask yourself where you feel whole and in what areas you feel as though some part of you is missing. It is by being fully present with what is happening—all aspects of it—that we begin to open to our inner wisdom and intuitive knowing about how to improve that area of our lives.

When we're out of our bodies with fear or caught in our minds trying to "figure it out" or "fix it", we do not have access to that inner wisdom. We just keep trying the same old things that have never worked for us before. We're stuck in a mental rut—a block.

To get out of the rut, we have to allow our energy to flow. That takes being fully present in our bodies while we face the issues of that area of our lives.

Facing our issues fully may be painful or embarrassing, but it's a necessary part of the balancing process. Once you see the issues properly and take suitable action to address them, a deep sense of fulfillment and satisfaction replaces the pain you feel and that area of your life comes naturally into balance.

Are you prepared to be truly honest with yourself? Are you prepared to take action to change your life? If so, here's how to restore balance in your life:

Exercise 8-2: Restoring Balance in Your Life

Have paper and pen handy to record notes.

1. Find a comfortable position and close your eyes.
2. Bring your attention to your breathing.
3. Take in a deep breath and let it out with a sigh. Repeat this 3 times.
4. Ground into the earth (see Exercise 5-5) and become fully present in your body and energy field.
5. Allow your awareness to tune into an area of your life that feels unfulfilled.

6. Do a check-in to explore how the situation in this area is affecting you physically, emotionally, mentally and spiritually.

7. Expand your awareness into the rest of your life. How is this situation is affecting your balance in other life areas?

8. Ask yourself the following questions:

   - Do I have all the facts of the situation that is causing me to feel unfulfilled in this area of my life? If not, how can I find out? Who can help me to understand what is really happening (for example, a therapist, an accountant, my doctor, my spouse)?

   - How am I personally contributing to the situation? How are my actions or avoidance making the situation worse?

   - If I could balance this area of my life, what would that look like physically, emotionally, mentally and spiritually?

   - What skills or knowledge would I need to achieve this balance? How can I obtain these skills or this knowledge?

   - How would I have to behave differently to move toward balance?

   - Am I willing to do what it takes to change the situation?

   - If so, what small step could I take right now?

9. When finished, take another deep breath and let it out with a sigh.

10. Open your eyes and make a note of what came up.

11. Then take action on that first small step and record what happens. This will guide you to the next step.

Summary

Our life chart is a snapshot of our life balance in the moment. It will change from day to day. Doing the chart weekly enables us to uncover the longer-term trends that may be developing in our lives. These trends are well worth exploring.

As we create new behaviors and choices that support wholeness, we find that our lives automatically balance around us. It seems like magic, but it's the natural outcome of allowing our energy to flow in alignment with who we truly are and what we truly want.

In the next chapter, we'll look at some frequently asked questions about managing energy in different situations.

CHAPTER 9

Questions and Answers

When people begin to learn about energy, questions often come up. In this chapter, we answer some of the questions our clients have put to us. We've grouped the questions under the relevant chapters for easy reference.

Questions on Chapter 1
The World of Energy

In Chapter 1, we learned how energy is a vital part of us and affects us in all areas of our lives. We discovered that most of us are already aware of energy at some level, and that we have "energy senses" that provide us with subtle information about our environment and interactions with other people. We also performed a variety of energy exercises to experience energy directly and consciously. The following are our responses to some of the questions people have asked us about the world of energy.

Q: Is there any scientific proof that subtle energy is real?

Yes. Many scientific studies have proven the reality of subtle energy and the effects of human energy on plants and objects. A full discussion is beyond the scope of this book. However, if you're interested in finding out more, we invite you to visit our website (energyisreal.com) where you'll find links to several scientific papers that describe subtle energy studies.

Q: If energy awareness is a natural part of us, why do most of us lose that awareness?

As children, many of us learned that what we were sensing didn't always correlate with what the adults in our lives were insisting was true. This is confusing for a child. We may have tried to ask questions about what we were experiencing, but because our parents had shut off their own sensitivity, they may have dismissed it as just an overactive imagination or may even have accused us of lying. And so for survival purposes we decided that it was easier and safer to ignore the information coming from our own energetic senses and to believe what the adults were saying instead.

Q: What about people who are highly sensitive? How did they develop their awareness?

Children are instinctively sensitive to energy. While a few highly sensitive people had supportive childhood environments that encouraged them to explore their energy senses, many energy-sensitive people had stressful home environments during childhood. They used their energy awareness to sense family members' emotional states. That way, they knew when it was safe to approach difficult family members and when it was best to avoid them. Eventually, they became highly sensitive to the slightest nuances so they could protect themselves in time.

Q: How does the news of large-scale catastrophes like wars, terrorist acts or natural disasters affect us? What can we do to protect ourselves energetically from their effects?

These events create an energy upset of global proportions that moves like a shock wave across the planet. If we take the time to notice our energy field, we can sense the impact.

When upsetting external events impinge on our fields, self-care is our top priority. We need to create safety first by getting grounded, becoming present and putting our bubble in place (See *Exercise 2-3: Creating an Energy Bubble Around You* on page 37.)

From that protective space inside our bubbles, we can pray or send love to the victims. If the love inside us inspires us to act, we can take suitable action to help. (Because fear or anger can distort our thinking, it's important that we feel love in our hearts before choosing what action to take.)

If the situation doesn't need any personal action from us, we can clear our fields of the upsetting energy, so it doesn't continue to affect us negatively for the rest of the day.

Questions on Chapter 2
Coming Home to Your Energy Self

In Chapter 2, we learned about the nature of our energy self. We also explored how we sometimes lose contact with that sense of self and then abandon our own needs, feelings, thoughts and values when dealing with others. We discovered how to bring our full awareness back into our bodies and energy fields and how to create a bubble of loving safety for ourselves within our energy. We also learned through direct experience how using our energy bubble helps us to stay calm and clear when dealing with stressful situations. The following are our responses to some of the questions people have asked about these topics.

Q: My bubble feels like a shield. How can I stay safe in relationships without pushing people away?

It's important to note that your energy affects other people, even when you're in your bubble. You are not separate. So even though you have the protective space of your bubble around you, your energy still affects others. When you're in calm, loving state, you'll evoke positive rather than negative reactions and behaviors from others. Because your energy feels safe to them, people will be more inclined to trust you and cooperate with you. So rather than pushing them away, your bubble actually helps you to communicate more easily with others.

Q: I'm shy, what can I do to feel comfortable meeting new people in a social situation?

First, ground to become present in your body. Then, create your bubble, feel the love in your heart and get in touch with that feeling of safety. The safety of your bubble will give you the courage to risk connecting with others. In addition, the loving energy within your bubble will help others to connect with you.

You may find that it helps to practice being in your bubble on your own first, using imagined scenarios of meeting people as described in *Exercise 2-4: Managing Your Boundary to Deal with People or Situations* on page 40. Once you're able to manage your bubble comfortably with these imagined scenarios then you can practice taking your bubble into real social situations.

Q: When my next-door neighbors fight, I feel stressed. What can I do?

Witnessing an argument or fight is energetically upsetting. It scares us and we become ungrounded because of what *they* are doing. We're letting others influence our thoughts and feelings.

Detach your thoughts from the negative details of your neighbors' argument. Ground yourself. Then create your energy bubble. Once you feel safe within, stay in your heart and try radiating love to those who are fighting. After they stop, make sure you clear your field of their negative emotional energy, using one of the clearing techniques on pages 121–126 in Chapter 5, *Maintaining Your*

Energy. That way, you won't carry their negative energy into your own life.

Q: When I stay as a guest in someone's home, I become forgetful and easily distracted. What can I do?

When we're a guest in someone's home, we're surrounded by their personal energies, as well as the energy environment of their home. We're in their territory, which makes us feel energetically uncomfortable. When this happens, we may move our energies partially out of our bodies. This can cause a "spaced out" or scattered feeling.

As guests, we also tend to behave on our hosts' terms. If we stay in this environment long enough, we can lose our sense of self. We may become robotic, like a child waiting to be told what to do. We may feel there is nowhere to go to be alone or we may tell ourselves, "Why be alone when I came to visit them?"

In a situation like this, immediately use the grounding technique (see *Exercise 5-5: Grounding* on page 104). That will bring your energies back into to your body.

Once you're present in your body, then you can create your bubble and connect with yourself (see *Exercise 2-3: Creating an Energy Bubble Around You* on page 37). This will give you the sense of safety you need to communicate authentically with your hosts or if needed, to create some time alone for yourself.

Q: What other benefits can I expect from using the energy bubble?

Here is what a client has to say:

"Personally, the energy bubble became a way of learning to take care of myself. Before I learned about the bubble, I found myself giving when I didn't really want to. I had a massive fear that nobody would like me, if I were honest with them and said 'No.'

"The bubble provided me with safe boundaries. It gave me the confidence to be more honest with myself and to know what I actually wanted, instead of worrying about what everyone else wanted around me.

"I had to spend some time alone to learn how to build that bubble, to discover what I liked and wanted and to become used to using my bubble to be around others. Once I learned how to do all this, then I became more honest about my needs. It made me confident enough to say this is what I want and this is what I want to do. And people still liked me!

"Now, I've become much more aware of my boundaries. When there's a conflict or issue in my life, it's not as severe as before. I don't experience dramatic highs and lows anymore, because things don't affect me in the old way."

Questions on Chapter 3
Becoming Clear Within

In Chapter 3, we explored our energy self in more detail and learned check-in techniques to tune into the innate wisdom available in the physical, emotional, mental and spiritual parts of our being. The following are our responses to some of the questions people have asked about these topics.

Q: When I try to do the emotional check-in, I don't get anything. How do I tune into my feelings?

If you're generally not aware of your feelings, you might be trying to tune into your emotional body from your intellect. Instead, try moving your awareness into your heart and then begin to tune into your emotions from there.

Tension can also interfere with your ability to sense emotions. If you're at work, you may not feel comfortable experiencing some emotions in the office environment. As a precaution before doing the emotional check-in, you might want to ensure that you're in a place where you can be alone with your feelings, without fear of disturbing others.

If you're already in a safe environment, for example working with an energy practitioner, sensing nothing can also be a sign there is some strong emotion coming up that you don't want to feel. When we're afraid, our energy contracts and this makes it harder to sense things. Take a few deep breaths to calm yourself and hold an attitude of gentle curiosity about what might be going on for you emotionally. Be willing to allow whatever you feel to come into your awareness. The best attitude when exploring your emotions is to view them without self-judgment. They are just a normal part of our energy.

Q: How can I speak my truth without upsetting other people?

If we really want to speak our truth, we need to first connect to our hearts. In any situation where we feel we need to speak up, the only truth that we can honestly share is our own experience and feelings. Nobody can argue with your feelings, because they just are what they are. The truth is not "You're hurting me." The truth is "I feel hurt right now" or "I need to feel heard, it's important to me." What you're feeling or needing is a valid truth.

When you speak the truth in that way, without blaming, then the other person can hear it without reacting defensively and you have a better chance of resolving the situation.

Before you decide to "speak your truth" to someone, do an emotional check-in (see *Exercise 3-2: Exploring Your Emotional Energy* on page 51) to find out your real feelings and what important need is not being met for you in the situation. Then go into your bubble to create safety for yourself and share your truth from your heart.

Q: Why should I make the Check-In Exercise a regular habit? Are there any real practical benefits?

The benefits become obvious when you experience it for yourself. Here is what one of our clients has to say about the benefits of using this skill regularly:

> *"Connecting with my energy self has taught me that I'm on a learning path. When I'm fully present and conscious with what is happening, I'm able to see the lesson that is facing me in my life. When I finally "get" it, I can feel results resonate within every cell of my being. Knowing I have this inner feedback mechanism, makes me feel freer to move forward in my life, confident that I'll be able to handle similar situations better in the future.*
>
> *"I have also learned that at the core of every challenge is some belief. I now do a spiritual check-in to examine whether my beliefs about a situation help me or make things worse. If my beliefs aren't serving me, I know that they are faulty and I can tune into my spiritual energy to show me a better solution to the problem. After practicing these skills for the last four years, my awareness now is at a completely different level from when I started this journey."*

- Another client shares the following experience:

> *"Having learned how to tune into the different levels of my energy, I now know how healthy energy flows in the body and I can tell the difference between healthy energy and nervous energy. The nervous energy feels more chaotic, like electrical static.*
>
> *"Being aware of when I'm mostly in my emotional body has helped almost every decision I've made. I ask myself, "Where am I now when I'm making this decision?" And even just recognizing in the moment*

that I'm mainly in my emotional or mental body, or have no awareness of my body, helps to make me more present. Then I take the next step to ground and restore my bubble before choosing what decision to make."

Questions on Chapter 4
Energy and Self-Care

In Chapter 4, we explored what stops us from doing our self-care and how that affects our energy levels. We also learned how to find out what self-care we need to keep our energies strong on all levels of our being—physically, emotionally, mentally and spiritually. The following are our responses to some of the questions people have asked about these topics.

Q: My life is so busy. How can I fit in regular self-care, as well as everything else I have to do?

Self-care is essential to help you to keep your energy strong throughout the day, so you can handle your other tasks efficiently and productively. While you may have to organize your day differently to make room for some self-care activities, it doesn't always have to take up a lot of your time.

In fact, there are often opportunities to incorporate self-care while you're doing other tasks. For example, at a meeting, you could drink plenty of water and breathe more deeply. Both of these actions would improve your brain functioning. You could choose to walk to work, or park your car a few blocks away from your destination and walk. You could run while taking the dog outside, or while pushing your child in a jogging stroller. You could choose to use the stairs, rather than take the elevator. You could pack yourself a healthy bag lunch or go to a vegetarian restaurant for a change.

These are only a few ideas to consider for improving your physical self-care. You'll find the best suggestions for you and your life will come from your energy self. Do a check-in at each level of your field (physical, emotional, mental and spiritual) and see what self-care you need right now (see *Exercise 4-1: Self-Care Check-In* on page 83).

Q: A week ago, I quit smoking and started eating lots of fresh vegetables, but now I have less energy than before I started. I thought self-care was supposed to make me feel better. What's going on?

When you quit a habit that was putting toxins in your body (like alcohol, drugs or smoking), your body will go through a detoxification stage. This is normal. It means your body is getting rid of the toxins and you're becoming healthier. However, detoxing often causes some unpleasant temporary withdrawal symptoms such as headaches, nausea, loss of appetite and fatigue.

Just make sure you drink plenty of fresh water to help your body to remove the toxins. And be especially kind to yourself by getting enough sleep, eating lightly, getting fresh air and so on. This will shorten the detoxing period and you'll soon feel great afterwards.

Q: I suffer from insomnia. Is there anything I can do energetically to get to sleep?

Insomnia typically occurs when our energy is overstimulated, rather than slowing down to prepare for sleep. It's helpful to do an energy check-in to discover whether the cause is physical, emotional, mental or spiritual.

An example of a physical cause is drinking caffeine too late in the evening or eating something that causes digestive distress. If this is causing your insomnia, then changing these evening habits will probably address the problem. If your body is feeling tense, then doing some stretching exercises should help to release the tension.

If the cause is emotional, for example feeling angry with someone, then you'll find that expressing the emotion in a safe way will help the energy to release and you'll feel sleepy soon afterwards. Journaling is very effective. Another way is to hit a pillow or yell into it. You can also stomp around, or even dance, to move the energy.

If your insomnia is caused by an overactive mind—perhaps you're reliving an argument or trying to solve some problem at work—go into your bubble and extend it to cover your whole bedroom. Then put the issue outside the bubble. Focus on your breathing and move your awareness into your body. Make your body comfortable, and think about the wonderful sensations of becoming drowsy and drifting gently off. Sleep should follow shortly.

Spiritual distress can also cause insomnia, for example because of an uncomfortable conscience or an important life issue that you're dealing with. If this is the case, use the bubble to help you to move to a more loving state and then let the love in your heart guide you to a solution. If nothing comes to you, put the issue outside your bubble and follow the same steps described earlier for preparing your mind and body for sleep.

Q: As a nurse in the emergency ward of a busy hospital, I deal with pain and trauma daily. How do I stay in my heart and do my job without burning out?

Compassion fatigue is a form of emotional burnout that is a frequent problem for emergency care workers. Self-care is a must to keep your energies strong. Low energy causes us to feel more vulnerable to the suffering of others and we can easily feel overwhelmed. We then find it necessary to close off our hearts to protect ourselves. While at work, make sure you take the necessary breaks for self-care and use your energy bubble to help you to stay in your heart. The loving energy within your field will help to calm you, as well as those in your care. It will also have a positive effect on your co-workers, improving morale and resulting in better treatment of patients.

Q: Can we use our energy to slow down or reverse the aging process?

Many of the signs and symptoms of aging result from inadequate self-care. This reduces our overall energy, causing tiredness and a reluctance to do exercise or take action. Being energetically run down affects such things as mental acuity, mood and motivation. This results in further decrease in our self-care and subsequently in our energy levels and health. We call it aging, but in truth, we've stopped looking after ourselves.

However, when we make a conscious choice to do what it takes to keep our energies strong and we follow up with loving self-care on all levels of our being, our energy and our bodies remain youthful and healthy. To reverse the signs of aging, besides proper self-care, we need to restore the healthy flow of energy in our bodies by addressing and clearing the energy blocks that we've built up over a lifetime. This typically takes the help of a body-centered therapist or an energy practitioner.

Q: Self-care seems like too much work. Why should I make the effort?

Here is what a client has to say about the benefit of self-care:

> "When I go out walking, it's time for ME. I'm present with myself when I am stretching my body outdoors. I don't care if I look silly. It's my life, my body and my well-being!"

Questions on Chapter 5
Maintaining Your Energy

In Chapter 5, we learned the basic energy management skills of conscious breathing, grounding, charging and clearing that we can use to build up our energies and to keep them strong throughout the day. The following are our responses to some of the questions people have asked about these topics.

Q. I'm under a lot of pressure at work. How can I manage my energy to avoid burnout?

It's important to know about the damaging effects of stress and burnout and to know the tools and techniques for reversing these effects. The dangers of burnout are many:

- **On the physical level**—Burnout puts extreme stress on your immune system, which leads to illness, stiffness and susceptibility to injury. You may feel physically exhausted. You may sleep a lot, but not feel rested. You may suffer from migraines. Adrenal exhaustion from stress may cause hormonal imbalances that affect the functioning of your thyroid.

- **On the emotional level**—You may feel you have nothing left to give in relationship. This dulls your sex drive and reduces passion. It can cause you to become critical of and irritated by loved ones, which can lead to resentment from your spouse or behavioral problems in your children. When you're burned out, there is a tendency to allow other people to make decisions for you. In excess, this can cause you to feel manipulated or victimized.

- **On the mental level**—Burnout causes confusion, leading to procrastination and poor decision-making. Loss of attention at work can cause costly mistakes and compromise your professional reputation. If you're a medical professional or an emergency worker, your burnout can endanger someone else's life. Inattention or confusion can also lead to accidents and injuries at home, at work or on the road.

- **On the spiritual level**—Burnout leads to negativity, pessimism and a failure to see positive solutions to problems. When burned out, you may begin to think in survival mode, causing self-absorbed isolation or rude and aggressive behavior towards others. In extreme cases, burnout can lead to depression or even suicidal despair, needing professional intervention or hospitalization.

You can avoid burnout if you know how to sense and manage your personal energy. Energy awareness enables you to catch any stresses in your life that need attention, before burnout happens. And it helps you to identify exactly where your life is out of balance.

Being able to manage your energy allows you to handle stressful situations easily and provides new energy to tackle the demands of your daily life. Practicing your energy management techniques can bring you back into balance before the stress overwhelms you. In addition, proper energy management allows you to handle situations in ways that actually reduce stress and lead to win-win situations for all parties.

To handle stress, the most powerful tools to use during your day are breathing, grounding and your energy bubble. Breathing helps to calm anxiety. Grounding gives you more energy and helps you to become present. And the bubble provides a sense of safety in your stressful work environment. When you leave work, make sure to clear your field before you get home so you're able to relax and enjoy the evening. This will enable your body and energy field to restore themselves and prevent burnout.

Q: I get panic attacks. What can I do to stop them?

When we experience a panic attack, we tend to move our energy partially out of our bodies. We feel paralyzed and unable to cope with the situation. To stop a panic attack, the best thing to do is to ground.

Grounding immediately brings your energy back into your body and gives you the presence of mind to create your energy bubble. Grounding also provides you with extra strength and energy.

Once you've grounded and created your energy bubble, you'll be able to decide how to deal with the situation.

Q: Traveling makes me nervous. Is there anything I can do energetically to feel more relaxed when I travel?

When we travel, we leave the safety of our home environment and enter the unknown. We find ourselves in the foreign territory of airports, hotels, train stations and even countries with different cultures and rules. We may feel helpless and at the mercy of the strangers we meet, including hotel clerks, taxi drivers, airline officials and fellow travelers. In addition, travel can result in unexpected experiences that cause us to feel even more threatened.

To be able to relax and enjoy traveling, it's important to stay connected with ourselves. The most important tools are grounding and breathing. Grounding enables us to become present in our bodies, while breathing, using the Complete Breath, helps us to calm down. Once we're present, we can use our energy bubble to create safety and to become clear about what action we need to take.

When we're able to keep our energy bubble in place while traveling, we find the loving energy that we hold in our bubble translates well into all languages and smoothes the way for our interactions with others.

When we see the world through loving eyes on our travels, we can't help but enjoy ourselves. Here is how Claudette manages her energy while traveling:

"I've traveled a lot in my life. The unknown is everywhere. From early on I learned to ground when something uncomfortable, unusual or unexpected would happen, because I didn't like feeling powerless in

those situations. I always went into my bubble to ask 'what can I do for myself right now, so I can feel safe?'

"Usually it was breathing that calmed me down. Then the answer would come to me to sit quietly and wait, or to go to talk to someone and ask questions. Grounding would give me the clarity to act in my best interest. Breathing helped me to focus on the NOW. This combination brought me the clarity to find the right action to take in any situation. Staying calm and not reacting to external influences, allowed me to find out what was going on internally. And I was always safe when I did that. Grounding also gives me extra energy, which I might otherwise waste in feeling panicky."

Q: I've heard I should ground when I meditate. How would that help me?

When people first learn to meditate, they often find it hard to stay focused. Their thoughts keep pulling them here and there. Grounding helps to calm the mind and to bring your energy fully into your body. You're then able to follow the breath and stay present. Here is one client's experience of using grounding in her meditation practice:

"In meditation, I used to be distracted by my mind, wondering whether I was balanced or aligned. Now, instead of thinking about alignment, I just feel for the energy movement and everything just clicks into place. I find that grounding sets me up for meditation more quickly, because it helps me to become present enough to sense how the energy moves in my body."

Questions on Chapter 6
Surfing Your Personal Energy Wave

In Chapter 6, we learned that our energy moves in cycles of expansion and contraction and we learned how to surf our personal energy wave successfully. The following are our responses to some of the questions people have asked about these topics.

Q: How do I know if what I'm experiencing is really a contraction and not depression or something else wrong with me?

The easiest test is to ask yourself if you had an expansion experience in the last day or so. If so, chances are that you're experiencing a contraction. Do *Exercise 6-1: Mapping Your Personal Energy Wave* on page 142 to confirm where you are on your energy wave. If you haven't had an expansion in a long while, you may not be in contraction. Consult with your doctor to find out what else might be causing your symptoms.

See also Chapter 7, *Restoring Inner Balance* for help on how to respond to the inner balancing messages that your symptoms may be giving you.

Q: I have to meet an urgent deadline, so I can't afford to take time off for contraction right now. How can I keep my energies expanded long enough to finish the job?

Because you're fighting what your energy naturally wants to do, you have to give yourself very good self-care to avoid energy depletion and prevent burnout. Use grounding, breathing with positive visualization and the charging exercises in Chapter 5, *Maintaining Your Energy*, to keep your energy strong during the project.

You'll probably experience a deeper contraction than normal later on, so make sure you give yourself time to contract after you meet your deadline.

Q: I've been working nonstop to meet this deadline for so many weeks; I have nothing left to give. What can I do to restore my energy?

If we continue to try to expand our energy and refuse to contract, eventually we're going to run out of energy and burn out. To recover, we consciously need to take the time to allow ourselves to contract.

Avoid heavy mental work. Instead, do such things as slow breathing, walking and engaging in quiet contemplation, preferably in nature. Allow thoughts and insights to arise naturally without strain or striving. Then record them. This is a time to reflect and learn from the past and allow new insights to come into your awareness.

Surrender to a deeper state of being. Feel the energy of your life force in your body and move your awareness into your cells. This will lead to physical renewal and healing.

Use the grounding and charging techniques in Chapter 5, *Maintaining Your Energy* to restore your energies more quickly. In the future, you can prevent burnout by paying better attention to your self-care and properly surfing your energy wave.

Questions on Chapter 7
Restoring Inner Balance

In Chapter 7, we learned how to use the clues provided by our energy self to decide what actions to take to return to inner balance quickly and easily. Here are our responses to some of the questions people have asked about these topics:

Q: How do energy blocks lead to disease?

To protect ourselves from reliving past hurts and traumas, we tend to avoid the part of the energy field where we store the memories of those events. When our energy is not there, the issues stored in that part of the energy field appear to "go away". That is, they subside out of our normal awareness. They have not really gone anywhere—we've just temporarily forgotten about them by moving our awareness elsewhere.

Awareness allows energy to move. Because we avoid being aware of the issue, the energy held in the affected part of the field can't flow and becomes "stuck" as an energetic block.

The physical body needs energy for health. Over time, an area that is energetically deprived or stagnant begins to break down physically. The underlying cells weaken and are not replaced as often. The surrounding tissues eventually become more susceptible to injury or disease.

Q: How do I heal my energy blocks?

To heal the physical condition fully, you must address and release the underlying emotional, mental or spiritual issue that is causing the condition. Use *Exercise 7-1: Restoring Your Physical Energy Balance* on page 149 to explore the issues that may be behind your physical symptoms. Then use Exercises 7-2 through 7-4 to balance your emotional, mental and spiritual energy while focusing on the part of your body where you hold those symptoms. This will help you to gain clarity on any emotional, mental or spiritual issues that may be associated with your physical condition.

Appendices A through D provide further help in interpreting what you discover. Becoming aware of the issue is often enough to shift a minor block. To clear more stubborn issues, you may need the help of a therapist or energy practitioner.

Once the underlying issue resolves, there is no longer a need to divert or repress energy in that area. The cells become properly nourished again and physical health returns.

Q: I worry about every little thing. How do I get my mind to stop worrying?

Constant worry can paralyze us from taking action in our lives, because we're afraid of making a mistake. When we do take action, we immediately worry about whether we did the right thing.

Worry shows a deep-seated lack of trust in ourselves, in others and in life itself. Worry is an unproductive mental habit that assumes the worst scenario will happen. In truth, our worst imaginings rarely happen and we end up wasting our precious life force by worrying needlessly.

A better use of our mental energy is to think about what we would rather have happen in our lives than what we fear. Because energy follows thought, it's important to choose consciously what you want to think about rather than letting your mind run wild with negative imaginings. You can treat worry as a message that is trying to get your attention about a potential negative situation. Give thanks for the message. Put your energy bubble in place and then decide if you need to take any action to prepare for or prevent the feared situation.

Also, consider what alternate scenarios might happen instead, that you would prefer. When you do this, your mind begins to think of creative ideas for making a better outcome unfold instead of the one you fear. As you take suitable action on those ideas, you'll find the future unfolds far more positively than you imagined. If you make a habit of responding creatively to situations in this way, you'll find yourself worrying less and enjoying life more.

Q: How do I deal with procrastination?

Almost all of us procrastinate from time to time. Usually it's because of fear and resistance. We may fear being overwhelmed. We may fear failure or even success if we worry that our success will cause us to have to make unwanted changes in our lives. As long as we procrastinate, fear keeps our minds closed.

To deal with procrastination, you need to face your fears honestly and courageously. In facing the fear, you deny the power of fear to stop you. In effect, you create the necessary courage to move forward in your thoughts. This forward motion then opens your mind to receive the necessary insights to resolve the issues causing your procrastination.

Because energy follows thought, we tend to draw to us what we focus on. If we focus on success, we become aware of all the associated insights, opportunities and help that will guide our way to success. If we focus on failure, we only notice those events, thoughts and reactions from others that reinforce our feelings of failure.

Once you've identified the fear that causes you to procrastinate, when that fear arises again simply notice that it's there. Then consciously visualize what you would prefer to happen, instead of what you fear. As you change your focus, you'll begin to feel motivated to start tackling the task that you were procrastinating.

Q. I'm tense all the time. What can I do energetically to get myself to relax?

First, do a physical check-in to see where in your body you're holding your tension. Then, do an emotional and mental check-in in that area of your body, to find out what underlying thoughts and emotions are creating the tension. Follow the instructions in Chapter 7, *Restoring Inner Balance* to restore balance emotionally or mentally. The physical body should relax naturally as a result.

Q: How can I be happy when I have so many problems in my life?

You can have problems and yet have happiness, too. Nothing needs to change in your external life for you to be happy—happiness truly is an inside job. To find happiness right now, regardless of what is happening in your life, follow the steps in Chapter 2, *Coming Home to Your Energy Self* to create your energy bubble and then put your problems outside the boundary.

As you radiate love into your energy field, you'll not only begin to feel happier, you'll also receive many creative insights for solving the issues in your life.

Q: How have your clients benefited from paying attention to the inner messages provided by their energy?

Here is what one client has to say:

"When I noticed myself looking to others for support and not getting it from them, I took this as a message to pay closer attention to my physical and emotional energy. As I explored what this pattern was about, I discovered that I tended to vent my anger on my friends, instead of addressing my problems directly with the person involved. I realized that venting wasn't the answer. It only kept me stuck in my painful emotions and did nothing to resolve the situation.

"By looking at my physical and emotional energy, I now know that I can gage my feelings based on how I'm reacting physically—especially how I'm breathing, where I breathe from or if I'm holding my breath. When I notice an emotional reaction forming and I take a deep breath before doing or saying anything, it gives me the time to think about how I want to respond to the situation, rather than reacting blindly."

Questions on Chapter 8
Energy and Your Life

In Chapter 8, we learned how to identify the places in our lives where we're not fully expressing ourselves, and we learned how to bring those areas back into balance. The following are our responses to some of the questions people have asked about these topics.

Q: At family gatherings, it's difficult for me to engage with anyone. Their conversation is full of small talk or people gossip about others. I feel empty and alone. What can I do?

When you're in a large group, and especially with family, it's important to get back to yourself and feel the love within you, rather than looking for it from others. Use grounding to become present in your body and energy field; then create your energy bubble. Feel the love inside your bubble and connect with the loving person that you are.

When you feel safer, try radiating the love inside you into the room. You'll uplift the energy in the room and everyone will benefit, including you. This will help you to feel more connected with others.

Q: As a new employee in an established company, I find it difficult to get the older employees to listen to my ideas for improving how we work. What can I do to get them to hear me?

When joining an established company whose members have been there for many years, newcomers sometimes feel it's hard to make an impact. They may feel the energy of the workplace is heavy and the old employees are too set in their ways about how things are done.

If you want to make changes, your best approach is to connect with the existing employees individually rather than as a group. Introduce yourself to each one and make an effort to get to know them better and learn about their interests. As they come to know you, your energy feels less threatening to them and you become less of an outsider. If you take the time to gain their trust and learn what is important to them, you'll be able to present your proposed changes in ways that are more likely to be supported. One of your new acquaintances may even step forward to champion your ideas to the rest of the group, which will further boost your chances of bringing in a change.

Q: What is the difference between love and caretaking?

Love is pure appreciation for another, delighting in them and their presence. Caretaking, on the other hand, involves assuming responsibility for another. We may do it in the name of love, but it's not by itself the same as loving.

Unless love accompanies the caretaking act, it's bound to lead to energetic depletion. Then we see caring for others as a form of self-sacrifice, which we believe necessary to prove our love. But if love is truly present, we've no need to prove it. We radiate our love without expectation or need.

The need to prove our love occurs only when we're not actually feeling loving. It covers up underlying feelings of resentment, anger, impatience or stress. Feeling guilty about these unloving feelings, we then feel driven to prove our love through self-sacrificing behaviors such as caretaking.

When we notice the theme of self-sacrifice in our lives, it's a message to learn how to care for ourselves. We can't truly love another while excluding ourselves from love.

Q: How can I use energy to attract abundance in my life?

Our state of abundance, or the lack of it, reflects how we regulate the flow of energy in and out of our lives. Wherever you feel "impoverished" in your life, whether it's in terms of time, love, beauty, play, creativity or money, tune into the innate wisdom of your energy self and ask what you need to come into balance.

Sense into who you really are and what longs for expression now. What experiences have you been holding back from yourself? If you could have or be anything at all, what would you most want right now? You'll receive the necessary impulses to come into balance—a thought, insight, hunch or just an inclination.

As you act on these impulses, you'll notice small signs of abundance start to occur in your life. Welcome these first tendrils of abundance moving towards you. Don't dismiss them as too small, or as "too little too late", but wholeheartedly delight in them and celebrate them! The energy of gratitude will magnify and accelerate the flow of abundance into your life.

Q. I feel blocked in expressing my creativity. What can I do to move forward again?

Do a mental check-in (see *Exercise 3-3: Exploring Your Mental Energy* on page 55) and see what you're telling yourself about your creativity. Chances are you're judging it or comparing yourself with others. The main reason people feel blocked is they've convinced themselves that they're not talented enough.

Perfectionism, self-judgment, fear of failure, a controlling attitude and fear of letting go are all ways that we limit our creative expression. Look at these issues as mental balancing messages and refer to *Appendix C: Mental Balancing Messages* for suggestions on how to deal with them.

If your problem is lack of inspiration, you need self-care on the spiritual level. Do *Exercise 4-1: Self-Care Check-In* on page 83 to find out what spiritual self-care you need right now.

Q: I have more than one passion in my life. Do I have to give up one passion to focus on the other?

You don't have to give up any of your passions. You can have all of them! You're only limited by how much time, energy and money you're able to spend on them.

Consider exploring whether there are ways of combining your passions in a synergistic way. For example, if you love music, but also long to become a psychologist, you could combine your passions by developing a form of music therapy. If you love sports and photography, becoming a sports photographer would be a natural combination.

Often when we have multiple passions, our energy self is telling us that our purpose involves combining them in creative ways. When we allow ourselves to do this, we find our lives take off in an exciting new direction.

Q. How do I find out what my purpose is?

To find your sense of purpose, it helps to do a spiritual check-in (see *Exercise 3-4: Exploring Your Spiritual Energy* on page 59) and notice what little longings stir your heart. Good clues pointing to your purpose are activities that give you joy, that you're naturally good at and that seem to be effortless for you.

If you follow up on those clues and pay attention to how your heart responds, you can find your way. When you follow up on a longing, if it leads to an expansion of the heart (felt as warmth and an increase of love for yourself and others) then you know that you're on the right track. If your action leads to a contraction of the heart, a sense of fear or dread, or coldness towards others, then you're drifting from your path. It's a simple guidance system, but well worth developing.

The heart uses the word "love" a lot. You might hear yourself saying, "I'd really love to do this", or "Do you know what I'd love to see?" or "I love that!" Pay attention to these messages. Follow what you love and your heart will guide you unerringly along your best path.

Q: How can managing my energy improve my life?

Here is what one of our clients has to say:

"I now realize the effects of harnessing my energy, rather than just reacting to the events and people in my life. I now consciously use my energy to focus on what I want to attract in my life. I'm more careful of where, when and how I put my energy out into the world, knowing that it affects my own life, the environment and other people.

"One of the most important skills for me is connecting to myself. Breathing and finding my center while using my bubble helps me to feel whole. It makes sure that I am present and aligned in body, emotions, mind and spirit. I can definitely feel the positive energy of my bubble affecting my life. I am more aware of how powerful I am in attracting what I want when I surround myself with positive energy."

Another client says:

"For me the most obvious benefit is that managing my energy helps me to settle my mind and stay calm in difficult situations. I typically do this by grounding and centering in my bubble. In that state, I reconnect with my true feelings about the situation and become fully conscious about what is happening. Recognizing my role in causing my problems gives me the power to let go of those behaviors that don't serve me in my life.

"For example, I recently chose to resign from my job. I was confused about how events unfolded and watched helplessly while what I'd gained in my career dwindled away. In trying to learn from this

experience, with Claudette's help, I connected with myself and heard the thought "I reached out and missed." I realized that I have a repeating pattern of self-sabotage in my life. When confronted by those in authority, I tend to leave the situation, rather than speak the truth. This pattern came from a childhood experience of feeling powerless against force of my father's opinions. I couldn't fight him, so I learned to walk away instead.

"In the safety of my bubble, I saw that I needed to trust myself enough to be able to have my feelings, while being tactful about sharing them with others. I also saw how I tend to take situations personally, which distorts my understanding of the bigger picture and triggers my old pattern of leaving in difficult situations.

"The key lesson my energy has taught me is to be aware of what is really happening and to consciously choose to respond in a positive way. I've learned not to keep myself small with disempowering behaviors, but rather to trust in the clarity and wisdom of my energy self. I've also learned that I'll continue to attract situations that allow me to grow and to learn from them. I now know that by opening my heart to let in the light of understanding and by feeling gratitude for each lesson, I can trust life to show me the way forward on my destined path."

Taking Your Energy into the World

Q: What can we do energetically to bring about peace, prosperity and wholeness to our planet?

The solution must begin with each individual. As you use energy consciously to improve your own life, you teach your children and loved ones by example. Children typically learn about energy quickly.

Your energy will also positively affect your friends, neighbors and co-workers. As they become curious about the results you're achieving in your life, encourage them to get their own copy of this book so they can experience the benefits of using these techniques for themselves.

We're all individually responsible for our own energy, but as others also learn how to manage theirs, a chain reaction will happen. More and more people will start to transform their energy and their lives. In this way, we can change the planet, one person at a time—beginning with ourselves.

Energy is real. When we all use our own energy consciously and wisely, together we will change the world.

Summary

The questions and answers in this chapter show many ways that we can use our energy consciously to make positive changes in our lives and to deal with daily life situations.

Of course, there is much more to the world of energy than we've been able to present in this book, and you may well have more questions that you'd like answered. We invite you to submit your questions to our blog where we'll do our best to address them for your benefit and that of other readers. You can access our blog from our website, energyisreal.com.

In the meantime, we encourage you to practice the energy management skills of centering, creating an energy bubble, conscious breathing, grounding, clearing and charging until you can do them easily.

One way to speed up this process is to associate a specific symbol or keyword for each technique every time you practice it. This will eventually condition your subconscious mind to create the associated energy state automatically, whenever you say the word or visualize the symbol that you used to anchor the skill.

For example, you could say the word "Ground!" or visualize the Earth every time you go through the steps of grounding into the Earth. You could say "Bubble!" each time you put your energy bubble in place. You can also use a gesture or unusual action, such as tugging your earlobe, to anchor the skill. With enough practice, you'll eventually be able to put your skills quickly into place whenever you need them.

If you practice using your energy awareness and the techniques in this book in your daily life, the benefits will soon be obvious to you. As your life begins to transform in positive ways, you'll discover that you can trust the wisdom of your energy self to guide you unerringly towards the path of your greatest joy and fulfillment.

For More Information

Website

If you would like further information about managing your energy, we offer additional tools and support on our website:

https://energyisreal.com

You can subscribe to our newsletter and follow links to scientific papers and other energy-related sites, read articles, download free tools, hints and tips, or check out our growing knowledgebase (FAQs).

For more experiential training, see our online event schedule listing the upcoming workshops, talks and teleseminars.

Join Our Facebook Group

We invite you to join our private Facebook community. We would love to hear how energy awareness has affected your life. It is also a great place to post questions. We can all learn much from one another and your experiences may be helpful to others.

Contact Information

CoreStar Publishing

email: contact_us@energyisreal.com

Website: https://energyisreal.com

Facebook group:

https://www.facebook.com/groups/energyisreal/

Appendices

- Appendix A: Physical Balancing Messages
- Appendix B: Emotional Balancing Messages
- Appendix C: Mental Balancing Messages
- Appendix D: Spiritual Balancing Messages

Appendix A: Physical Balancing Messages

The following table describes some common examples of physical balancing messages and explains what they may mean. Bear in mind that only you know what life imbalance is causing your particular physical problem. Check into your own energy field and pay attention to the insights available to you there.

Accidents

Cause:	Accidents may result from physical balance problems, visual or hearing problems or from inattentiveness—for example, when we're distracted by something else going on in our lives.
Message:	"Pay attention"
	An accident can be a subconscious way to get attention from others or from ourselves. A serious accident is often a "wake-up call" to pay attention to how we're living our lives. It may be that we're ignoring the promptings of our conscience, or the accident may be providing a convenient way out of a situation that we don't like. Whatever the reason, the accident is telling you that you need to pay closer attention to the self. This is a call to be fully present in your body and in your life.
How to Respond:	Connect with yourself and do a check-in to find out what may be causing the problem and how to deal with it. (See Chapter 7, *Restoring Inner Balance* for instructions on how to do this.)

Addictions

Cause | The underlying motive in all addictions is a positive one—to comfort the self. Unfortunately, addictions provide only temporary relief, because they just deal with the outer symptoms (discomfort) of the problem. They don't resolve the underlying causes, such as chemical dependency, emotional pain, low self-esteem, loneliness, boredom or despair. Eventually, addictions create more stress, because of their frequently toxic effects on our bodies and minds. We end up making poor decisions under their influence, which causes further upsets in our lives.

Message: | "You need self-care."

How to Respond: | It's not easy to break the repetitive cycle of addiction, but with determination, commitment, and practice it can be done. A full discussion on the healing of addictions is beyond the scope of this book. However, there are some things you can do for yourself energetically that will help.

Whenever you feel the addictive urge, immediately ground into the earth (see *Exercise 5-5: Grounding* on page 104) and create your energy bubble (see *Exercise 2-3: Creating an Energy Bubble Around You* on page 37).

Next, place the object of your addictive desire outside the bubble (see Exercise 2-4: Managing Your Boundary to Deal with People or Situations on page 40). In the safety of your bubble, do a check-in to find out what healthy self-care you really need right now (see *Exercise 4-1: Self-Care Check-In* on page 83) and give that to yourself. This technique works well for milder addictions, such as caffeine, tobacco, sugar or shopping.

For more serious addictions, it is best to seek professional help. If you're dealing with drug or alcohol abuse, for example, you may need to undergo a medically-supervised detoxification program. A therapist or energy practitioner can help you to clear the underlying psychological issues that are triggering your addiction. A 12-step recovery program, such as Alcoholics Anonymous, or Al-Anon can also provide very effective support on your healing journey.

Chronic Illness

Cause: Chronic illness occurs when we block the flow of energy in our bodies. Typically, this occurs where we hold fear. It can also point to a place where we hold unpleasant thoughts, emotions, memories or traumas. We tend to move our energy away from the area to avoid feeling the unpleasantness.

Over time, the underlying cells of the body starve and weaken from lack of energy. When this happens, the associated part of the body becomes more susceptible to injury or illness.

Message: "A change is needed."
This is a message to deal with the underlying emotional, mental or spiritual issues that you're repressing in that area of your body. You may have some long-standing beliefs that limit you—fear of moving forward, for example. Or you might be in a toxic environment

(emotionally or physically), which you need to leave. It's causing you harm to stay there.

How to Respond: Do a self-care check-in to explore the physical, emotional, mental and spiritual issues you may be holding in the location of the illness. (See *Exercise 4-1: Self-Care Check-In* on page 83 for instructions.) Then follow through on any self-care insights you may receive for your healing. You can also check Appendices B, C and D for more help with the emotional, mental or spiritual issues that you uncover during your check-in.

Fatigue or Weakness

Cause: Fatigue or weakness is a sign of energy depletion. There are many things that can drain our energy, including:

- **Physical causes**—hunger, thirst, lack of sleep, poor nutrition or illness

- **Emotional causes**—grief, guilt, remorse or fear

- **Mental causes**—mental burnout, overwork, feeling overwhelmed or self-judgment

- **Spiritual causes**—depression, despair, lack of purpose, loss of faith or compassion fatigue

Fatigue or weakness can also occur when we're experiencing an energy contraction or when we're healing after an illness, surgery or a deep spiritual transformation.

Message: "It is time for self-care."

How to Respond: Do a check-in to find out what physical, emotional, mental or spiritual self-care you need to restore your energy (see *Exercise 4-1: Self-Care Check-In* on page 83).

Then, follow through with appropriate self-care in that part of your energy. If you're in the contraction phase of your energy cycle, see Chapter 6, *Surfing Your Personal Energy Wave* for how to deal with it.

Food Cravings

Cause: Food cravings can have a hormonal basis, such as those experienced during pregnancy. They may also be a reaction to a vitamin or mineral deficiency. For example, a calcium deficiency can trigger a craving for cheese or chocolate.

Food cravings can also have an emotional basis. For example, we may be craving comfort or more enjoyment in our lives and use food as an easy way to provide this for ourselves. A food craving may also be an escape from taking action. Or it can be the way that we comfort ourselves when under stress.

Message: "A real need is not being met."

How to Respond: Do a check-in to find out where you might be failing to meet your real needs on the physical, emotional, mental or spiritual levels of your being (see *Exercise 4-1: Self-Care Check-In* on page 83). If you think your cravings may be hormonal, ask your doctor about this. See also "Addictions" on page 236.

Internal Temperature Changes

Cause: If we suddenly feel too hot or cold, regardless of the temperature in the room, it may be due to metabolic, hormonal or emotional causes. For example:
- Feeling hot can result from not drinking enough water (dehydration), a menopausal hot flush, adrenal stress or by experiencing embarrassment or anger.
- Feeling cold can result from hunger, fatigue, poor thyroid function or by experiencing fear or terror.

Message: "Check your self-care."

How to Respond: This may be a reminder to look at your level of self-care. Explore further. Have you missed a meal or hormonal supplement lately? Are you dehydrated? If you have a fever or other symptoms of illness, consult your doctor.

If you suspect the cause is emotional, do an emotional check-in (see Exercise 3-2: Exploring Your Emotional Energy on page 51) to find out what emotion may be behind your symptom. Then see *Appendix B: Emotional Balancing Messages* for details on how to deal with the underlying emotion that you discover.

Joint Problems

Cause: Joint problems can result from under- or overuse of the affected joint. Typically, we leak energy from the joint area.

Message: "What are you avoiding?"

Energy leaks are a way of diverting energy away from something. The affected area may hold memories of an emotional or physical trauma (accident or surgery) that you don't want to feel.

How to Respond: Do a check-in to explore the physical, emotional, mental and spiritual issues you may be holding in the affected area (see *Exercise 3-5: Exploring How Your Energies Interact* on page 62.) If you uncover a traumatic memory in the joint area, an energy practitioner can help clear the trauma and repair the energy field to support the healing process.

Pain (Acute)

Cause: Acute pain can result from physical injury, gastric upset, strain or disease. It can also result from severe emotional distress, such as the sudden loss of a loved one—this can make us feel like we've been punched in the stomach or as if our hearts are tearing apart.

Message: "Get help!"
Acute pain is your body's urgent cry for help—it is impossible to ignore.

How to Respond: Do a check-in to find out if the cause is physical or emotional (see *Exercise 4-1: Self-Care Check-In* on page 83). If you feel the cause may be physical, consult your doctor.

If the pain is sudden and disabling, consider it a potentially life-threatening emergency. Call an ambulance or get someone to take you to the nearest hospital. It may be a false alarm, but it's better to find out for sure, rather than to risk your life by delaying.

If you suspect an emotional shock is the cause of your pain, first see your doctor to make sure there is no physical problem and then seek professional counseling for emotional guidance and support.

Pain (Chronic)

Cause: Chronic pain occurs in those places where our energy flow is weak or disconnected, often at the site of an old injury or operation in that area.

We tend to avoid using the part of the body where we feel pain. This aggravates the problem, because avoidance directs energy away from the area, weakening it further.

Message: "You need to reclaim a part of yourself."

How to Respond: When we divert our attention away from a painful area, we're effectively cutting off part of ourselves, including all the associated emotions, thoughts, memories and beliefs that we hold there. To restore wholeness, we need to reconnect with our energy self in the parts of the body that we have been avoiding.

Our painful places hold much valuable information for our healing. Becoming present with your pain allows that healing information into your awareness and helps to relieve the pain.

Use *Exercise 3-5: Exploring How Your Energies*

Appendix A: Physical Balancing Messages 243

Interact on page 62 to uncover what emotional, mental or spiritual messages your pain might be trying to tell you. Then refer to Appendix B, C or D for details on how to deal with the underlying emotion, thought or belief that you discover.

Pain (Unexplained)

Cause: Pain can occur even when there is no obvious physical problem. This is often labeled "psychosomatic pain".

Message: "Something is amiss emotionally, mentally or spiritually."

How to Respond: Do a check-in for your emotional, mental and spiritual energy in the location where you feel the pain (See *Exercise 3-5: Exploring How Your Energies Interact* on page 62.) Then refer to Appendix B, C or D for details on how to deal with the underlying emotion, thought or belief that you discover.

Stiffness

Cause: Muscle stiffness can mean pooling of energy or lymph (from lack of exercise) or lactic acid buildup (from recent strenuous exercise). (For joint stiffness because of arthritis, see "Chronic Illness" in this table.)

Message: "Move or stretch"

How to Respond: If the problem is over-exercising, causing a lactic acid buildup, gentle stretching and massage will help to clear the buildup. If the stiffness is due to lack of exercise leading to pooling of blood or lymph, take it as a message that you need more physical movement. Do a self-care check-in to find out what particular self-care you need right now (see *Exercise 4-1: Self-Care Check-In* on page 83.) Also, consult your doctor about what activities are safe for you to begin at your current level of health and fitness. Then see a qualified personal trainer or physiotherapist to develop the right exercise program for your body and condition.

Tension

Cause: Typically, tension is caused by fear or anxiety. (See also "Fear and Anxiety" in *Appendix B: Emotional Balancing Messages*)

Message: "You're afraid that something painful or unpleasant is about to happen."

How to Respond: For temporary relief, techniques such as conscious breathing (see the Complete Breath on page 93), grounding (see page 104) and the energy bubble (see page 37) will help to reduce anxiety and physical tension.

For a more permanent solution, you need to resolve the impending problem or release the fear and the beliefs causing it. Do an emotional, mental and spiritual check-in around the tension (See *Exercise 3-5: Exploring How Your Energies Interact* on page 62.) Then refer to Appendix B, C or D for details on how to deal with the underlying emotion, thought, or belief that you discover.

Appendix B: Emotional Balancing Messages

Emotions tell us about the power balance in our lives. We need to pay attention to them. The following table describes some common examples of emotional balancing messages and explains what they may mean:

Anger

Cause:	Anger arises when someone or something disappoints or threatens us and we feel a strong need to take action. We might want to confront, argue, fight, complain or report them to the authorities. Either way our energy will not allow us to stand passively by.
Message:	"Take constructive action to resolve this situation."

How to Respond:	Anger when properly expressed is a positive agent for change. Make sure you have the correct facts before acting.
	  Check with the other person to ensure you haven't misinterpreted their behavior.
	  Go into your bubble to become clear about what is upsetting you and what action to take (see *Exercise 2-3: Creating an Energy Bubble Around You* on page 37). You may need to take a brisk walk, raise your voice or simply speak your needs in a clear and strong way.
	  Once you've taken the needed action, the energy releases and the pressure is gone. Typically, the situation causing the anger resolves itself once you feel heard or

take positive action.

Depression

Cause: Depression is a sense of helplessness and hopelessness. We may feel like victims in our lives.

Depression often results from repressing anger or other powerful emotions. This deadens all our feelings, including the positive ones.

Message: "Reclaim your emotions to reclaim your power."

How to Respond: To lift depression quickly, it helps to do physical movement or exercise, for example, go for a brisk walk or dance to some lively music. This is a temporary solution that works well for mild depression.

For serious or chronic depression, it's best to seek professional help to explore the emotions and beliefs giving rise to the pattern. Work with a body-centered psychotherapist or energy practitioner to release your held emotions in a safe environment. This will give you some temporary relief.

The next step in healing depression is to clear the beliefs causing your sense of helplessness. This will prepare you for the final step—learning to reclaim the power in your life. Again, a therapist or energy practitioner can help you with these steps. (See also "Anger" on page 245.)

Envy

Cause: This emotion arises when we wish that we had something that someone else has.

Message: "You want this too! Start to make plans to bring it into your life."

How to Respond: Envy points to where you haven't been developing your own gifts and abilities. When you're envious of others who have achieved something, you can take it as a message that you need to do the same, not to compete, but for your own happiness. You need to allow your own potential gifts and abilities to unfold in their unique way.

Do a spiritual check-in (*Exercise 3-4: Exploring Your Spiritual Energy* on page 59) to find out what unique dreams, interests or talents you're longing to bring forward in your life. Then take the first small step towards expressing them.

Fear or Anxiety

Cause: Fear or anxiety occurs when we expect a painful experience or a threat to our survival.

Message: "Be prepared."

How to Respond: If it's something you've no control over, do what you can to prepare as best you can and then let go. For example, you're afraid of flying, but need to visit another country. You take the precautions of selecting the safest airline, choosing the seat beside the emergency exit, taking out flight insurance and making sure your will is up to date. Having done all you can do, you must now put your trust in the pilot and cabin crew to get you safely to your destination. This part is out of your hands, so it's time to let go and surrender. Maybe even try to enjoy the flight!

If your fear or anxiety is chronic, an early childhood trauma may be affecting you subconsciously. Consult a therapist or energy practitioner to help you explore and release the subconscious patterns causing your fears.

Grief

Cause: Grief is a feeling of overwhelming loss. We can feel grief for the loss of a loved one, when we lose a part of the body (through accident or surgery) or go through a change of life. We can also feel bereaved when we move to a new country, leave home (homesick), or when we retire from a profession that we loved and identified with most of our lives.

Message: "Be with your self."

You've identified so completely with what you've lost that you don't know who you are anymore. You've lost contact with yourself.

How to Respond: Grief can open the heart if you let it. Don't allow yourself to shut down or become bitter or resentful about your loss. Resolve instead to feel the grief and let it move as an energy wave through you.

It takes time for grief to heal. When the sense of loss changes into gratitude and peace, then you'll know you're ready to move forward in your life.

If you have difficulty dealing with grief, you may find it helpful to join a bereavement support group or work with a therapist who specializes in grief and loss. An energy practitioner can also help you to move the heavy energy of grief from your heart and to reconnect with yourself.

Guilt

Cause: Guilt is the discomfort we feel when we've violated one of our own rules or are acting contrary to our conscience.

Guilt can be a useful message if the rule or belief is valid—then guilt serves to remind us when we stray from our integrity. However, if the rule or belief is something we learned in childhood that no longer makes sense to us as adults, then the guilt is a neurotic pattern that inhibits the expression of our natural abilities and creativity.

Message: "You've broken an important rule."

How to Respond: Do a spiritual check-in (see *Exercise 3-4: Exploring Your Spiritual Energy* on page 59) to examine the rule or belief that is causing the guilt. Does it still make sense for you? If so, take action to correct the situation about which your conscience is warning you.

If the rule or belief causing the guilt is no longer valid, then consider seeing an energy practitioner or therapist who can help you to access and reprogram the subconscious. Effective therapies include Brennan Healing Science, Neuro-Linguistic Programming (NLP), hypnotherapy and Emotional Freedom Technique (EFT).

Hatred

Cause: This powerful emotion arises when we dislike someone so intensely that we go to extremes to avoid them or to shut them out of our lives. We may have once loved them, but experienced some perceived betrayal that we're unable to forgive. In extreme cases, hatred can cause a desire to harm the other person or to seek revenge.

Message: "You're giving your personal power away to another."

How to Respond: Hatred makes us feel like victims. When we make others responsible for our unhappiness, we give away our power to them. To reclaim your power, let go of blaming others and take what steps you can to improve your own life. See *Exercise 8-2: Restoring Balance in Your Life* on page 190 to explore how you can create a healthy, balanced and fulfilling life for yourself.

If you're having trouble letting go of blame or hatred, consult a therapist or energy practitioner to help you to reclaim your power.

Hurt or Disappointment

Cause: Feeling hurt or disappointed happens when an expectation hasn't been met and we're interpreting it as a rejection of our worth.

Message: "Change your expectations or approach."
Detach your worth from the situation. Treat it simply as an event you need to deal with. The old approach is not

	working.
How to Respond:	Do a spiritual energy check-in to access creative solutions to the situation. (See *Exercise 3-4: Exploring Your Spiritual Energy* on page 59.)

Jealousy

Cause:	This emotion occurs when we believe there is not enough of something (e.g. love, money, success or fame) to go round and feel we must fight to get or keep our share. We may need to control possessions, situations or other people to maintain the status quo.
Message:	"You're holding on too tightly" You're relying on the external (other people and things) to make you happy.
How to Respond:	Instead of focusing on what you can get from others or from the situation, shift your focus to what you can give—not from a sense of duty or exchange, but from the sheer pleasure of generosity. Do a spiritual check-in (see *Exercise 3-4: Exploring Your Spiritual Energy* on page 59) to find a dream, a cause or a longing that moves you to contribute or give of yourself to others. Taking action towards a cherished dream will build your self-worth and lead you towards real happiness.

Remorse

Cause: This emotion occurs when we feel guilty about our past actions and wish that we had done things differently. We're unable to forgive ourselves for what happened. We're stuck in a mire of guilt and constantly reliving it only sinks us deeper.

Message: "Make amends."

How to Respond: Take action to resolve the situation and make amends as best you can, for example:

- **Apologize**—It's never too late to tell the injured party that you're sorry. If they are deceased, offer a prayer to them with your sincere apology or send a letter to their family.
- **Make amends**—Perform an act of good faith to help or honor the injured party. Ask them how you can make amends and try your best to undo the damage you caused them.
- **Forgive yourself**—Forgive yourself and resolve to behave more wisely in the future. Wish the injured party well and move on with your life.

Resentment

Cause: Resentment occurs when we feel angry about a situation, but powerless to change it. It leads to blaming others for our unhappiness and to feeling victimized.

Because we don't act to change the situation, the anger behind our resentment is unable to resolve itself and the energy stagnates.

Message: "Let go of the past."

Resentment is a killer—this energy can eventually lead to serious illness if not dealt with. Don't let it continue to fester.

How to Respond: Do an emotional check-in to connect with the anger underlying your resentment (see *Exercise 3-2: Exploring Your Emotional Energy* on page 51). See what actions you need to take to resolve the situation that's causing your resentment. Take the necessary action, then let the past go and become responsible for your own happiness. (See also "Anger" on page 245.)

Sadness or Longing

Cause: Sadness occurs when we passively wish for something more or different from what we have now.

Message: "Do your part to make it happen."

How to Respond: Pay attention to what you miss or long for. It is showing you how your life could be better. Then take steps to create that in your life.

If your sadness is because you miss or long for a particular person who is unavailable, then notice what traits you especially like in them and see what you need to do to develop those traits in yourself.

Appendix C: Mental Balancing Messages

The following table describes what some of the most common mental balancing messages mean and what action typically helps to restore balance.

Apathy

Cause:	Apathy is a sense of not caring about anything. ("Whatever. Do what you want, I don't care.") This may result from emotional or mental burnout, for example, over-giving in relationship or overwork. Another cause is being overwhelmed after a powerful physical or emotional shock, a devastating loss or a failure in something we once cared deeply about. Apathy can also occur when we have given our power away to someone else, for example, when we feel helpless in a situation over which they have control.
Message:	"You need self-care."
How to Respond:	If you're suffering from burnout or shock, do a check-in to find out what self-care you need right now to restore your energies (see *Exercise 4-1: Self-Care Check-In* on page 83). If you've experienced a disappointing setback or failure, or if you've given away your power, go into your bubble and reconnect with yourself. Ask yourself what you really want and need in this situation and take suitable action (see *Exercise 2-3: Creating an Energy Bubble Around*

You on page 37.)

Confusion

Cause: We become confused when we can't understand a situation and don't know how to deal with it. For example, we may be sensing something intuitively that we can't explain rationally. Or we may be in a new situation, where our old information, rules and behaviors no longer apply.

Mental confusion can also occur when our physical energy is low (because of illness or fatigue) and our brains are no longer functioning optimally.

Message: "Seek guidance."

How to Respond: The message here is to access the "big picture" for more general information on the situation. This may involve doing some research or getting training. Find an experienced mentor or teacher to help you to learn the necessary new skills.

If you're dealing with the irrational or the unknown, go into your bubble and reconnect with your spiritual energy to access your inner wisdom.

If confusion is because of energy depletion, self-care will restore your energies and help you to think more clearly. Do a check-in to find out what self-care you need right now. (See *Exercise 4-1: Self-Care Check-In* on page 83.)

Indecision

Cause: Indecision occurs when we're afraid of making the wrong choice. We may be using a limited either/or scenario, failing to see there may be other choices that could work better for all concerned.

Message: "What does your heart want?"

You're trying to make a decision purely from your intellect, but your heart has other ideas. In order to make a confident decision, your mind and heart must agree.

How to Respond: Go into your bubble and connect with your heart (see *Exercise 2-3: Creating an Energy Bubble Around You* on page 37). Looking at the situation from this more loving perspective, see what other choices exist that would bring your heart and mind into agreement. Choose the option that creates a win-win solution for all parties. Let yourself be creative!

Inertia (Feeling Stuck)

Cause: Inertia is a state where we want to curl up and disappear or do nothing. It is a form of escape from reality.

We feel stuck when we've become locked into old behaviors and habits and are afraid to change. We may feel like we're running on a treadmill or that we're trapped in a situation with no way out.

Message: "You're in a rut and have stopped growing."

How to Respond: Make a small change anyway and see what happens!

Any change, no matter how small, will interrupt the mind pattern that says, "I can't" or "I won't." If you catch yourself saying, "I can't" to yourself, use a positive affirmation instead. For example, change "I can't dance" to "I dance effortlessly".

Laughter and silliness are also great antidotes to fear. For example, try singing "I can't" or "I won't" in an operatic voice. That will usually break the rut and pull you in new directions.

If you still have trouble, consider seeing a therapist or energy practitioner who can help you to clear the subconscious programming that is keeping you stuck. Effective therapies include Brennan Healing Science, Neuro-Linguistic Programming (NLP), hypnotherapy and Emotional Freedom Technique (EFT).

Mental Overwhelm

Cause:	Mental overwhelm occurs when too many issues are competing for our attention. Or we may be trying to do more than we can handle in the moment.
Message:	"You need to prioritize."
How to Respond:	Go into your energy bubble (see *Exercise 2-3: Creating an Energy Bubble Around You* on page 37) and connect with yourself. This will give you clarity. Make a list of everything that needs your attention. Then prioritize the items in order of urgency and importance. For each high priority item, find some step that you can easily do, however small (for example, look up a phone number).

That one step leads to the next, and the next and the next, until you make it.

All great achievements start with a single small step, followed by another. There is always something you can do towards your goal. Find the smallest step and do it.

Mind Chatter

Cause: Mind chatter is a running commentary inside our heads, usually negative or self-critical, that keeps us feeling trapped and distracted.

Message: "Your energy is caught in your head."

How to Respond: Breathe deeply and focus your awareness on the breath (see *Exercise 5-2: The Calming Breath* on page 95.) This will bring you back into the rest of your body and calm the mind. Grounding (see *Exercise 5-5: Grounding* on page 104) and using your energy bubble (see *Exercise 2-3: Creating an Energy Bubble Around You* on page 37) will also help.

Perfectionism

Cause: Perfectionism occurs when we're driven by details and trying to meet impossibly high standards. It often results in delays and lateness.

We may be trying to prove our worth to someone (or ourselves.) Or we may be afraid of failure or rejection. Perfectionism may also be an attempt to control or create order in our environment, especially if we're feeling threatened by chaos or confusion in some other area of our lives.

Message: "You've lost yourself."

In striving for perfection, you've lost sight of what is truly important.

How to Respond: Go into your bubble and reconnect with your own heart and spirit. Take the time to explore who you really are and what you really care about.

From this deeper perspective, look at how perfectionism affects your life. Ask yourself if there are better and more life-enhancing ways to accomplish your goals. Try doing things differently and be willing to learn from each experiment.

If you can't let go of your perfectionism, do a spiritual check-in to explore the beliefs and issues underlying your behavior (see *Exercise 3-4: Exploring Your Spiritual Energy* on page 59). To change deeply embedded beliefs, consider seeing a therapist or energy practitioner who can help you to reprogram the subconscious. Effective therapies include Brennan Healing Science, Neuro-Linguistic Programming (NLP), hypnotherapy and Emotional Freedom Technique (EFT).

Procrastination

Cause: Procrastination occurs when we put off taking action on an ever-growing pile of to-do's. We may take action only on unimportant activities, rather than tackling the high-priority ones. Procrastination is often a form of resistance.

Appendix C: Mental Balancing Messages

	If prolonged, procrastination leads to overwhelm.
Message:	"You're bullying yourself."
How to Respond:	Chances are, there are some self-critical or "should" thoughts in your head that are tyrannizing you. Shifting to kindness helps to shift the energy. Tell yourself, "C'mon let's ..." For example, "C'mon let's make that phone call now." (See also "Mental Overwhelm", "Resistance" and "Inertia" in this table.)

Resistance

Cause:	Resistance is a refusal to take action even though we know we need to. We refuse because we're afraid of pain, failure or facing the unknown. For example, we resist going to see a doctor, because we're afraid to hear the diagnosis. Or we resist going to relationship counseling, because we don't want to admit our relationship is failing. Resistance can also appear as boredom, inability to concentrate or procrastination. We use any excuse to avoid doing what we're supposed to do.
Message	"Face your fear."
How to Respond:	When we face our fears head-on, we find the courage to act. Go into your bubble to create a feeling of safety for yourself (see *Exercise 2-3: Creating an Energy Bubble Around You* on page 37.) This will help you to become clear about the situation and about what you fear. While in your bubble, do a self-care check-in to find out

what you need to help you move forward in this situation. (See *Exercise 4-1: Self-Care Check-In* on page 83. See also "Fear or Anxiety" in *Appendix B: Emotional Balancing Messages*.)

Worry

Cause: Worry results from obsessing over an imagined future problem for ourselves or loved ones.

Worry has been called "interest paid on trouble before it is due".

Message: "Focus on what you DO want."

How to Respond: Most of our worries never actually happen. We've wasted our energy and created unnecessary stress for our loved ones and ourselves.

It is better to make use of the energy law "energy follows thought" to visualize what you would prefer to have happen, instead of what you fear. Visualizing what you want focuses the mind on solutions and creative possibilities. Options will occur to you that you might have missed while obsessing over imagined threats.

You can then make conscious choices that will help the preferred outcome to happen. (See also "Fear or Anxiety" in *Appendix B: Emotional Balancing Messages*.)

Appendix D: Spiritual Balancing Messages

The following table describes some of the most common balancing messages at the spiritual energy level and what action you might need to take to come into balance.

Blocked Creativity

Cause:	Things that can block our creativity include: • Self-criticism • Perfectionism • Fear of failure (or success) • Lack of confidence Children are naturally creative. When insensitive adults judge or ridicule our early creative attempts, the pain of that experience blocks us from expressing our creative energy. Later in life, we may believe that we're not creative and have no talent.
Message:	"Let yourself play!"
How to Respond:	Creativity thrives in a playful environment. Give yourself time to develop and explore your skills. Let yourself become a beginner or an experimenter. Creativity is a never-ending exploration. There is no such thing as perfection, failure or success—only opportunities to have fun with new creations and ideas. See Chapter 8, *Energy and Your Life* to learn more about how to stimulate your creativity. To release deeply embedded creative blocks, consider seeing a therapist or energy practitioner who can help

you to clear childhood fears about creative expression.

Effective therapies include Brennan Healing Science, Neuro-Linguistic Programming (NLP), hypnotherapy and Emotional Freedom Technique (EFT).

Boredom

Cause: Boredom results from blocking our self-expression and creativity. As children, we may have been discouraged, criticized or punished for our high spirits. As a result, we may have decided that it wasn't safe to risk expressing ourselves. When we squelch our self-expression and creativity, we lose our sense of excitement and passion for life. Boredom is also a sign that our life is not in balance.

Message: "It's okay to be you."

How to Respond: Do a spiritual check-in (see *Exercise 3-4: Exploring Your Spiritual Energy* on page 59) to find out who you really are and to reconnect with your innermost passion.

Also, look at your life balance chart (see *Exercise 8-1: Your Life Balance Chart* on page 185) and see in which life areas you may be wasting energy that could be used in more fulfilling ways. Then follow the steps in *Exercise 8-2: Restoring Balance in Your Life* on page 190 to improve the quality of your life.

Controlling Behavior

Cause: Controlling behavior occurs when we're afraid that we won't get what we want, so we try to make it happen. It arises from a lack of trust in others to give us what we need. We also try to manage our environment, or those around us, so we can feel safe.

Message: "Let go so you can receive."

How to Respond: Most people are happy to help. However, when we try to micromanage a situation and the behavior of others, we energetically repel the very support and love that we want. As a result, we have to do everything for ourselves. It is only when we surrender control that we learn that support is there for us.

Go into your bubble and place the situation and the other people concerned outside of it. Surrender to the loving energy in your bubble, allowing it to calm you and give you clarity on what action to take, if any. See *Exercise 2-4: Managing Your Boundary to Deal with People or Situations* on page 40 for details on how to do this.

If controlling behavior is a recurring problem in your life, consider seeing a therapist or energy practitioner to help you to clear the subconscious programming that prevents you from trusting that support is available in your life.

Despair

Cause: Despair occurs when we've given up hope and can't see any way out of our problems.

Message: "Connect with your spirit"
You need some "big picture guidance" from your own spirit to help steer you in the right direction.

How to Respond: Do a spiritual check-in to access your inner wisdom so you can make the right decisions for your life. See *Exercise 3-4: Exploring Your Spiritual Energy* on page 59 for instructions on how to do this.

Extreme Materialism

Cause: This condition occurs when we try to fill a sense of inner emptiness with material possessions. But no matter how many things we amass, it doesn't help. And eventually it leads to a sense of despair.

Message: "You're thirsting for a deeper sense of self"

How to Respond: You can only fill your inner emptiness with your own spirit. Do a spiritual check-in to connect with your spiritual energy (see *Exercise 3-4: Exploring Your Spiritual Energy* on page 59) and explore what you need in your life to feel more fulfilled.

Feeling Lost or Helpless

Cause:	We feel lost or helpless when we've lost connection with ourselves. We may have allowed others' demands to override our own needs so often that we don't know what we want or who we are anymore.
Message:	"Connect with yourself."
How to Respond:	You've lost your sense of self and need to reclaim your safe space. Go into your bubble (see *Exercise 2-3: Creating an Energy Bubble Around You* on page 37) and reconnect with who you really are and what you really need in this situation.

Feeling Unwanted or Excluded (Always an Outsider)

Cause:	The cause of this particular symptom typically lies in your childhood experiences. If your mother didn't want a child or if you felt no one had time for you growing up—this can leave a lifelong subconscious imprint of feeling rejected and unwanted. Feeling like an outsider causes us to hang back from getting involved in groups, fearing rejection. Others may interpret our aloofness as an insult or as a wish to be left alone, so they may ignore or reject us, which fulfills our worst fears.
Message:	"Welcome others into your life" Risk rejection and try to connect with others anyway. Be the first to welcome them into your life.

How to Respond:	Use the energy bubble (see *Exercise 2-3: Creating an Energy Bubble Around You* on page 37) to create safety for yourself and then take the initiative to create group activities that you can enjoy with others. The safety of your bubble will give you the courage to risk connecting with others. In addition, the loving energy within your bubble will help others to connect with you. You may find that it helps to practice being in your bubble on your own first, using imagined scenarios of meeting people as described in *Exercise 2-4: Managing Your Boundary to Deal with People or Situations* on page 40. Once you're able to manage your bubble comfortably with these imagined scenarios then you can practice taking your bubble into real social situations. Treat people as you would like them to treat you, with a warm welcome, and you become an insider automatically.

Feeling Wrong or Bad

Cause:	Feeling we're always in the wrong or intrinsically bad, occurs when we allow the opinions of others to become more important than the truth of who we are. We may have no sense of our own power and may feel like a victim when we're with others.
Message:	"Manage your boundaries"
How to Respond:	Use your energy bubble to manage your boundaries around other people (see *Exercise 2-4: Managing Your Boundary to Deal with People or Situations* on page 40.)

Lack of Abundance

Cause: Many things can cause a lack of abundance, including:
- Lack of self-worth—"I don't deserve it."
- Belief that scarcity is the norm—"Money doesn't grow on trees"
- Pride—"I don't want your charity!"
- Victim or childish attitudes—"They won't let me have it."
- Belief that money is bad— "Money is the root of all evil"
- Belief that money is unspiritual—"It is harder for a rich man to enter the Kingdom of Heaven…"

Message: "Your beliefs are blocking abundance."

How to Respond: Do a spiritual check-in (see *Exercise 3-4: Exploring Your Spiritual Energy* on page 59) to discover what limited beliefs may be keeping you in scarcity and to open to creative ideas for changing your situation. See also Chapter 8, *Energy and Your Life* for other techniques to improve the Abundance sector of your life.

Learning Disability

Cause: We repeatedly make the same mistakes without learning from them. A learning disability may have psychological or perceptual causes.

A psychological learning disability may occur if our parents didn't listen to us, devalued our ideas and imposed their opinions on us. This creates a subconscious need to assert our own views or knowledge to prove that we exist and that our opinions are important. However, identifying too strongly with our own knowledge or opinions can make us feel threatened when anything contradicts them, because it calls our very sense of self into question. To protect that sense of self, we may resist new information. This creates a learning disability, for it's only by assimilating new information that we learn.

A learning disability may also result from a perceptual problem such as dyslexia, which, when we were children, made it hard to understand what we were being taught. Adults may have labeled us as stupid or slow. If we believed them, our belief that we're stupid will block our ability to learn. We'll give up easily and won't even try.

Message: "Notice the patterns."

Repeating patterns are clues to where you may hold outdated opinions or knowledge about yourself.

How to Respond: Do a spiritual check-in to explore the repeating patterns in your life and see what you can learn from them. What alternate choices could you make in these situations that you haven't tried yet?

If you think that you may be dyslexic, consider having yourself tested. There are unique programs available today to help dyslexics of any age overcome their perceptual difficulties and learn normally.

Life Feels Meaningless

Cause:	This condition occurs when you have no sense of purpose guiding your life. It can happen when you ignore the promptings of your heart because they appear impractical or if you abandoned a cherished childhood dream to please someone else. For example, you really wanted to be an artist, but your parents discouraged you, so you studied business instead.
Message	"Connect with your heart's longing."
How to Respond:	First, connect with yourself—do a check-in for your spiritual energy and open to sensing what longings you hold in your heart for your life (see *Exercise 3-4: Exploring Your Spiritual Energy* on page 59). These longings are the key to your purpose. Then, sense what small action you can take now towards bringing your heart's dream into reality. Following these two steps will infuse you with purpose and fill you with the energy and enthusiasm to make the necessary changes in your life.

Resignation

Cause:	Resignation occurs when we give up out of a feeling of futility or helplessness.
Message:	"Are you really powerless in this situation?"
How to Respond:	If you surrender to someone whose demands are harmful to you because you're afraid to stand up to them, then

you're abandoning yourself—you're escaping from your own responsibility and power. You need to reconnect with yourself to look for better choices than the limited options given by the other person.

Use your bubble to create safety and clarity for yourself (see *Exercise 2-3: Creating an Energy Bubble Around You* on page 37). Then from this new perspective look at what other options might be available to you. (See also *Exercise 2-4: Managing Your Boundary to Deal with People or Situations* on page 40.)

Spiritual Longing

Cause:	This occurs when we yearn for more fulfillment in our lives. Ignoring our spiritual longings can lead to a deep sense of sorrow and can make our lives feel meaningless. When we look to others to fulfill our lives for us, we place a heavy burden on our relationships. They can't fulfill our longing, no matter how hard they try.
Message:	"Find your true purpose." Only by following our true purpose can we find the sense of completion and fulfillment we seek.
How to Respond:	Do a spiritual check-in (see *Exercise 3-4: Exploring Your Spiritual Energy* on page 59) to find out what life path excites you and what steps you can take towards it.

Appendix D: Spiritual Balancing Messages

Superiority or Self-righteousness

Cause: A superior or self-righteous attitude typically masks a secret fear that we're inferior or unworthy (bad).

It may also mask a fear of needing others. Judging others as inferior or bad is a way of rejecting them before they can reject you. In effect, it's saying, "Who needs you. I can do it myself."

Message: "Go inside to discover your true worth."

When you feel safe inside, there is no longer any need to judge or reject others.

How to Respond: Go into your bubble and connect with your self to feel the true safety and value of your being (see *Exercise 2-3: Creating an Energy Bubble Around You* on page 37).

From this place of inner safety and wholeness, you'll be able to meet others as equals, resulting in richer and more rewarding relationships.

Index

A

Accidents, 235
Acute pain, 241
Addictions, 170, 236
Aging, 207
Anger, 245
Anxiety, 247
Apathy, 255
Aura. *See* Energy field.
Aura Brushing exercise
 alone, 122
 with a partner, 123

B

Balancing messages
 emotional, 150, 152, 245–53
 mental, 156, 255–62
 physical, 146, 147, 235–44
 spiritual, 159, 160, 263–73
Basic Charging technique, 112
Becoming present
 in body, 31
 in energy field, 33
Blocked creativity, 159, 224, 263
Boredom, 264
Boundary
 changing, 23
 creating safety, 36
 exercises, 39
 managing around others, 39
 reaction to threats, 36
Breathing exercises
 Calming Breath, 94
 Cleansing Breath, 96
 Complete Breath, 92
 with visualization, 97

Burnout
 dangers of, 208
 recovering from, 214
 symptoms of, 208

C

Centering, 31, 229
 while interacting with others, 38
Charging exercises
 Basic Charging, 112
 Color Breathing, 113
Charging the energy field
 benefits of, 111
 how to, 112
 when to, 117
Check-In exercise
 emotional energy, 51
 mental energy, 55
 physical energy, 47
 questions and answers, 200
 restoring life balance, 189
 spiritual energy, 58
Chronic illness, 237, 242
Chronic pain, 242
Clearing
 home environment, 125
 how to, 119
 reasons for, 118
 when to, 127
Clearing exercises
 Aura Brushing, 122
 Aura Brushing with a Partner, 123
 Clearing Environmental Energies, 125
 Waterfall Cleanse, 120

Color Breathing technique, 113
Compassion fatigue, 206
Confusion, 256
Conscious breathing
   benefits of, 91
   Calming Breath exercise, 94
   Cleansing Breath exercise, 96
   Complete Breath exercise, 92
   with visualization, 97
Contraction phase
   resisting, 136
   surfing, 138
Controlling, 265

D

Depression, 213, 246
Despair, 50, 266
Detoxification self-care, 204
Disappointment, 250

E

Emotional energy, 50
   balancing messages, 150, 152, 245–53
   blocks, 66
   check-in examples, 52
   check-in exercise, 51
   imbalances
      causes of, 150
   repression, 66
   restoring balance, 152
   self-care, 77, 81
Energy
   basic laws of, 89
   benefits of managing, 7
   clothing and objects, 6
   environmental, 5, 125
   group, 4
   human, 3
   questions and answers, 193
   types of
      emotional, 50
      mental, 53
      physical, 47
      spiritual, 57
Energy awareness
   conscious use of, 15
   importance of, 7

life balance, 171, 189
   questions and answers, 193
Energy blocks
   causes, 64, 215
   healing, 216
Energy bubble
   creating, 36
   questions and answers, 196
   use of, 196
Energy cycles
   exercise to map your cycle, 141
   questions and answers, 213
   resisting, 135, 136
   surfing, 133, 137, 138
Energy field
   boundary, 20
   defined, 20
   sensing, 20
Energy interaction
   exercise to explore, 62
Energy laws, 89
Energy maintenance
   questions and answers, 208
   suggested daily routine, 128
   tools, 91
Energy repression
   causes, 64
   emotional, 66
   mental, 68
   physical, 65
   spiritual, 69
Energy self, xv, 43, 44, 53, 56, 60, 61, 62, 64, 70, 145, 162, 200, 202, 204, 215, 223, 225, 227, 229
   connecting with, 31
   effect of losing connection with, 30
   questions and answers, 196
Energy senses
   exercises to explore, 17
   types of, 13
Envy, 247
Expansion phase
   resisting, 135
   surfing, 137

F

Fatigue, 238
Fear, 247
Feeling hurt, 250
Feeling lost, 267
Feeling stuck, 257
Feeling unwanted or excluded, 267
Feeling wrong or bad, 268
Food cravings, 239

G

Grief, 248
Grounding
  benefits of, 101
  definition, 101
  how to, 103
  questions and answers, 208
  when to, 107
  while meditating, 212
Grounding exercises
  basic technique, 103
  with a partner, 105
Guilt, 249

H

Hatred, 250
Helplessness, 267

I

Indecision, 257
Inertia, 261
Insomnia, 205
Internal temperature changes, 240

J

Jealousy, 251
Joint problems, 240

L

Lack of abundance, 269
Learning disability, 269
Life balance
  abundance, 174, 223
  career, 182
  communication, 174
  health, 178
  home and family, 176
  learning, 181
  leisure and social life, 182
  passion, 180, 224
  play and creativity, 177, 224
  problems, 168, 170
  purpose, 184, 225
  questions and answers, 220
  relationship with self, 173
  relationships, 179
  restoring, 171, 189
  role of energy awareness, 167
Life balance chart
  analyzing, 186
  exercise, 184
Longing, 253
Love and caretaking, 222

M

Managing energy
  at work, 221
  during medical emergencies, 109
  for global peace, 227
  in dangerous situations, 109
  in social situations, 198, 221
  making a complaint, 107
  telephone calls, 107
  to attract abundance, 223
  to avoid burnout, 208
  while driving, 110
  while traveling, 108, 211
Mapping your personal energy wave, 141
Materialism, 266
Meaninglessness, 271
Mental energy, 53
  balancing messages, 156, 255–62
  blocks, 68
  check-in examples, 56
  check-in exercise, 55
  repression, 68
  restoring balance, 157
  self-care, 78, 81
Mental energy imbalances
  causes of, 156

Mental overwhelm, 258
Mind chatter, 259

P

Pain
    acute, 241
    chronic, 242
    unexplained, 243
Panic attacks, 210
Passion, 179
Perfectionism, 224, 259, 263
Personal energy wave. See Energy cycles
Physical energy, 47
    balancing messages, 146, 147, 235–44
    blocks, 65
    check-in examples, 49
    check-in exercise, 47
    repression, 65
    restoring balance, 148
    self-care, 77, 80
Physical energy imbalances
    causes of, 146
Procrastination, 218, 260

R

Real self. See Energy self.
Remorse, 252
Resentment, 252
Resistance, 261
Resisting contraction, 136
Resisting expansion, 135

S

Sadness, 253
Self-care
    aging, 207
    benefits of more energy, 80, 81
    best approach, 82
    caretaking others, 222
    compassion fatigue, 206
    detoxification, 204
    effects of neglecting, 77, 78
    emotional, 77, 81
    importance, 79
    insomnia, 205
    mental, 78, 81
    physical, 77, 80
    questions and answers, 203
    reasons for neglecting, 74
    spiritual, 78, 81
Self-righteousness, 273
Sensing energy
    boundaries of other people, 24
    energy radar, 15
    places and objects, 26
    questions and answers, 193
Speaking truth, 201
    questions and answers, 200
Spiritual energy, 57
    balancing messages, 159, 160, 263–73
    blocks, 69
    check-in examples, 60
    check-in exercise, 58
    repression, 69
    restoring balance, 160
    self-care, 78, 81
Spiritual energy imbalances
    causes of, 159
Spiritual longing, 272
Stiffness, 243
Superiority, 273
Surfing your personal energy wave
    contraction phase, 138
    expansion phase, 137
Surrender, 215, 271

T

Tension, 200, 244
Types of energy
    emotional, 50
    interaction between, 61
    mental, 53
    physical, 47
    spiritual, 57

U

Unbalanced life
    causes of, 168
    restoring balance, 171, 189
    symptoms of, 170

Unexplained pain, 243
Ungroundedness
   effects of, 101, 102
Unwanted energies
   clearing, 118
   effects, 118
45

W

Waterfall Cleanse exercise, 120
Weakness, 238
Worry, 217, 262

About the Authors

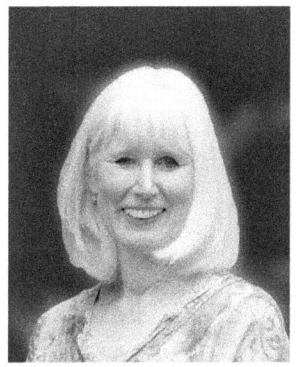

Gail Christel Behrend is an engineer, teacher, writer, and speaker. In addition to developing training courses for corporate clients, she has also been an energy practitioner for over 20 years. Gail is a graduate of the Barbara Brennan School of Healing in Miami, Florida, and is a certified Infinite Possibilities trainer. She resides in Vancouver, BC Canada.

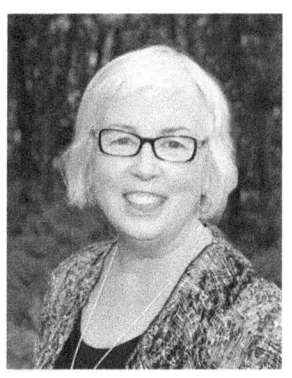

Claudette Anna Bouchard is a speaker, writer, mentor and life energy coach. A graduate of the School of Energy Mastery in Sedona, Arizona, she has over 30 years' experience as an energy consultant with clients throughout Asia, Europe and North America. Claudette is also certified by the Conscious Dying Institute in Boulder, Colorado as an end-of-life doula/coach and instructor. She resides with her husband in Vernon, BC Canada.

Both authors offer personal energy training to individuals and businesses. For more information, visit our website: **https://energyisreal.com**.

www.ingramcontent.com/pod-product-compliance
Lightning Source LLC
Chambersburg PA
CBHW060457090426
42735CB00011B/2021